SIMPLIFIED

EXAM FOR THE CERTIFICATION
OF PHARMACY TECHNICIANS
STUDY GUIDE

By
David A Heckman, PharmD

DISCLAIMERS & COPYRIGHT

ExCPT® Exam Simplified: Exam for the Certification of Pharmacy Technicians Study Guide

ISBN-13: 978-1942682035
ISBN-10: 1942682034

ExCPT® is a registered trademark of the Medical Certification Institute, Inc. ExCPT® Exam Simplified is not affiliated with or endorsed by the Medical Certification Institute or the National Healthcareer Association (NHA).

The author does not assume and hereby disclaims any liability to any party for losses, damages, and/or failures resulting from an error or omission, regardless of cause.

This publication is not a substitute for medical advice. For medical advice, consult a medical professional.

This publication is not a substitute for legal advice. For legal advice, consult a legal professional.

This publication does not contain actual exam questions.

Copyright © 2015, 2016 by David A. Heckman
All rights reserved. This book is protected by copyright. No portion of this book can be reproduced in any form, including mechanical or electronic reproduction, without express written permission from the author.

Book cover design by Keeling Design & Media, Inc.

Published by Heckman Media

Printed in the United States of America

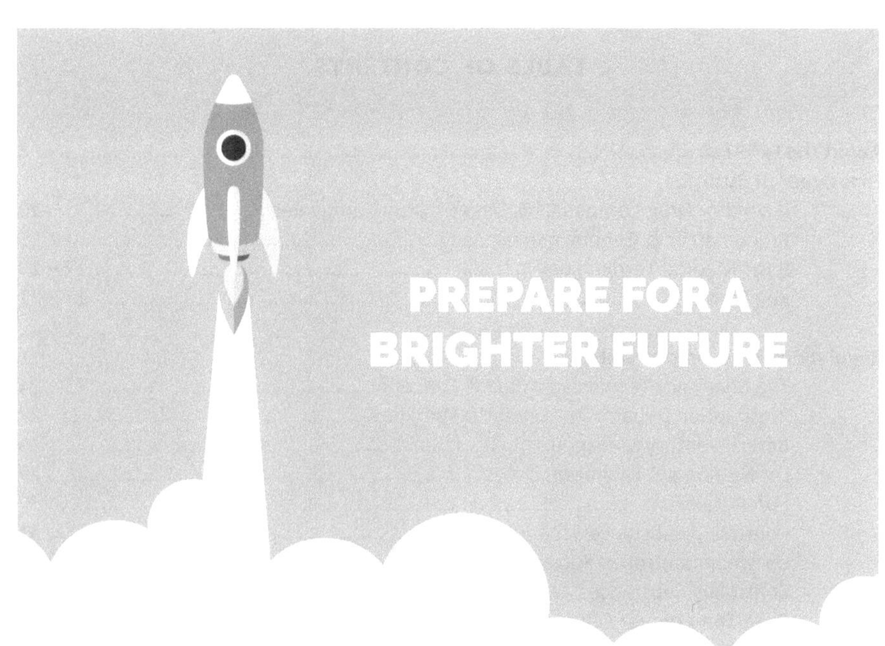

CPhT /// ACADEMY

100% ONLINE ExCPT EXAM PREP

presented by David A Heckman, PharmD

LAUNCHING JANUARY 31, 2016

Only at

www.CPhTAcademy.com

TABLE OF CONTENTS

TABLE OF CONTENTS

ABOUT THE ExCPT

- Exam for the Certification of Pharmacy Technicians (ExCPT)
- Register at www.NHAnow.com
- Exam registration fee: $105
- Exam must be taken within 6 months of registration
- Exam is administered at PSI Testing Centers
- Computer-based exam
- 120 multiple-choice questions
- Questions assess knowledge and skills related to the following areas:
    - Regulations & technician duties
    - Drugs & drug therapy
    - Dispensing process
- Approximately 30% of the questions involve critical thinking
- 2 hours and 10 minutes to complete
- To pass, the examinee must earn a scaled score of 390 out of a possible 500

FIRST ORDER OF BUSINESS
Get You Up to Speed

Before we begin reviewing the material outlined on the ExCPT exam blueprint, we need to bring everyone up to speed with some background information. This portion of the study guide will be especially helpful for those of whom have little to no prior pharmacy experience. We will explain brand (innovator) vs generic drug companies, brand vs generic drug names, basic medical terminology, and some key terms and concepts. Let's get started!

INNOVATOR DRUG COMPANIES & GENERIC DRUG COMPANIES

There are two types of drug companies - innovator drug companies and generic_drug companies. Innovator drug companies are heavily involved in drug discovery research and clinical trials to determine the safety and effectiveness of potential new drugs. Discovering a new drug that is both safe and effective is challenging. Less than one-tenth of one percent of new drugs are able to gain FDA approval and reach the market. When an innovator drug company discovers a potential new drug, they file a patent and then attempts to prove that the drug is safe and effective. Under this patent, the innovator drug company has the exclusive right to manufacture the drug (no other drug company can copy their idea) for about 20 years, until the patent expires. To protect their idea, these drug companies usually file a patent several years before clinical trials begin. Normally, it takes 10 to 13 years after a drug is discovered before the FDA finally approves a new drug (that is, *if* it gains FDA approval). By the time a new drug reaches the market, most innovator drug companies only have 7 to 10 years remaining on the patent. During this time, innovator drug companies must charge high prices to recoup the expenses accumulated from years of research & development, including all of the research that went into products that failed to gain FDA approval. Once the patent expires, generic drug companies begin selling their own copy of the drug. Since generic drug companies do not have the expenses associated with new drug discovery, they are able to offer a lower price compared to innovator drug companies.

Note: Occasionally, a patient will want to know when a brand product will be available generically. This is difficult to predict. Innovator drug companies frequently hire lawyers to acquire patent term extensions.

INNOVATOR DRUG COMPANY EXAMPLES

Merck & Co.
Johnson & Johnson
Eli Lilly
Pfizer
GlaxoSmithKline
Abbott
Amgen
Roche
Sanofi
AstraZeneca

GENERIC DRUG COMPANY EXAMPLES

Mylan
Actavis
TEVA
Sandoz
Watson
Greenstone
Hospira
Apotex
Dr. Reddy's
Mallinckrodt
Lupin
Par

BRAND NAMES & GENERIC NAMES

You will need to know both the generic name and brand name for the most commonly prescribed drugs. This is because healthcare professionals and patients often use brand names and generic names interchangeably.

Generic Names – the name of the active ingredient. In the US, the United States Adopted Names Council (USAN) is responsible for assigning generic drug names. The USAN is involved to reduce the chance that a new drug will receive a name similar to one or more drugs that are already available on the market. It is important that drug names are unique to prevent mistakes by prescribers and misinterpretation of prescriptions by pharmacists and pharmacy technicians. A synonym for the "generic name" is the "established name."

Brand Names – the company that discovers a new drug (the innovator drug company) chooses the brand name for that drug. During the time when a drug is under patent, the innovator drug company has the exclusive right to produce that drug, as we discussed on the previous page. After the patent expires, the innovator drug company may continue to produce the brand product, but generic drug manufacturers can legally produce and sell a generic equivalent version as well. Generic drug companies usually name their version of the product by the generic name, but, in some cases, they create a new brand name. This is why we sometimes see drugs with two or more brand names. Synonyms for "brand name" include "trade name" and "proprietary name."

BASIC MEDICAL TERMINOLOGY

Most English medical terms are combinations of Greek or Latin prefixes, root words, and/or suffixes. For this reason, it is in your best interest to learn the meaning of the Greek and Latin word parts we most commonly see in English medical terms. See charts below.

Word Root	Meaning	Example
Andr(o)-	Man	Androgen
Angi(o)-	Blood vessel	Angina
Arter(i)-	Artery	Arteriole
Arthr-	Joint	Arthroscopic surgery
Bio-	Life	Biohazard
Brady-	Slow	Bradycardia
Bucc-	Cheek	Buccal lozenge
Carcin-	Cancerous	Carcinoma
Cardi-	Heart	Cardiologist
Derm-	Skin	Dermatologist
Enter-	Intestines	Enteric-coated tablets
Gastr-	Stomach	Gastroesophageal reflux
Gen(esis)	Produce, generate	Genetic
Gluco-	Sweet	Glucose
Glyc-	Sugar	Hyperglycemia
Isch-	Restriction	Ischemic heart disease
Hem(at)-	Blood	Hematology
Hepat-	Liver	Hepatoma
Lip(o)-	Fat	Liposuction
My(o)-	Muscle	Myelitis
Narc(o)-	Numb, stupor	Narcotic
Nas(o)-	Nose	Nasal spray
Nephr-	Kidney	Nephrology
Neur-	Nerve	Neurology
Ocul-	Eye	Ocular
Onc-	Tumor	Oncology
Ophthalm-	Eye	Ophthalmology
Oste-	Bone	Osteomyelitis
Ot-	Ear	Otic
Path-	Disease	Pathology
Pharmaco-	Drug	Pharmacotherapy
Phren-	The mind	Schizophrenic
Plasia-	Development	Hyperplasia
Poro-	Porous	Osteoporosis
Proct(o)-	Anus, rectum	Proctologist
Psych-	Mind	Psychosis
Pyr(o)-	Fever	Antipyretic
Ren-	Kidney	Renal
Rhin-	Nose	Allergic rhinitis
Schiz(o)-	Split	Schizoid
Scler-	Hard	Atherosclerosis
Tachy-	Fast	Tachycardia
Thromb-	Clot	Thrombosis
Ur-	Urine	Nocturia
Vas(o)-	Blood vessel	Vasodilation

Prefix	Meaning	Example
Ante-	Before	Ante room
Anti-	Against, opposed to	Antiepileptic
Di-	Two	Dihydrogen monoxide
Heter(o)-	Different	Heterogeneous
Hom(o)-	Same	Homogeneous
Hyper-	Over, above	Hypertension
Hyp(o)-	Under, below	Hypotension
Micro-	Millionth	Microgram
Milli-	Thousandth	Milligram
Mono-	Single, one	Monoxide
Poly-	Many	Polypharmacy
Post-	After	Post-traumatic stress

Suffix	Meaning	Example
-al	Pertaining to	Intestinal
-algia	Pain	Myalgia
-ase	Enzyme	HMG CoA Reductase
-asis	Condition	Psoriasis
-emia	Blood condition	Leukemia
-emesis	Vomiting	Hyperemesis
-ia	State, condition	Hypokalemia
-iac	Pertaining to	Cardiac
-ic	Pertaining to	Prostatic hyperplasia
-ical	Pertaining to	Biological
-ion	Process	Dilution
-ism	Process, condition	Hypothyroidism
-itis	Inflammation	Arthritis
-lepsy	Attack, seizure	Epilepsy
-logy	The study of	Anesthesiology
-oid	Resembling	Opioid
-oma	Tumor	Sarcoma
-ose	Carbohydrate	Sucrose
-osis	Abnormal condition	Ketoacidosis
-ous	Pertaining to	Gangrenous
-penia	Deficiency	Leukopenia
-rrhea	Discharge	Diarrhea
-rrhage	Burst, excessive flow	Hemorrhage
-tension	Pressure	Hypertension
-tensive	Pressure	Hypotensive
-tic	Pertaining to	Neurotic

KEY TERMS

Absorption – the movement of a drug from a delivery medium (e.g. tablet, capsule, transdermal patch) into the bloodstream.

Acute – a sudden or rapidly occurring symptom or condition, usually of an urgent nature. Opposite of chronic.

ADME – an acronym that stands for "Absorption, Distribution, Metabolism, and Elimination." This describes the order by which drugs enter and exit the body.

Adrenal Gland – an anatomical structure located above each kidney that secretes several hormones, including cortisol, aldosterone, epinephrine, and norepinephrine.

Adrenergic – pertaining to neurons that release epinephrine or norepinephrine. Epinephrine and norepinephrine are associated with the fight or flight response.

Agonist – a substance that stimulates an action. For example, adrenaline (or "epinephrine") is an alpha and beta-receptor agonist. By stimulating these receptors, adrenaline elevates heart rate and blood pressure.

Analgesic – a substance or drug that reduces pain.

Anaphylaxis – a severe, potentially life threatening allergic reaction.

Anesthetic – a substance or drug that induces partial or complete loss of sensation.

Angina – severe chest pain caused by insufficient blood flow to the heart.

Angiotensin Converting Enzyme – a key catalyst within the body that is involved in the production and release of blood pressure-raising hormones.

Antacid – a substance or drug that neutralizes stomach acid.

Antagonist – a substance or drug that opposes an action. For example, metoprolol is a beta-receptor antagonist ("beta blocker"). Metoprolol interferes with the stimulation of beta-receptors, thereby opposing increases in heart rate and blood pressure.

Ante Area – the space directly adjacent to the clean room. The air quality in the ante area should be at least ISO class 8 (see "ISO classification" for more details).

Antiarrhythmic – a substance or drug that prevents and/or treats cardiac arrhythmias.

Antibiotic – a substance or drug that kills or opposes the reproduction of microorganisms.

Anticholinergic – a substance or drug that opposes parasympathetic nervous system activity. The parasympathetic nervous system is associated with rest & digestion.

Anticoagulant – a substance or drug that delays and/or prevents blood clotting.

Anticonvulsant – a substance or medication that prevents and/or treats seizures.

Antidepressant – a substance or drug that prevents and/or treats mental depression.

Antidiabetic – a substance or drug that lowers blood sugar levels.

Antidiarrheal – a substance or drug that prevents and/or treats diarrhea.

Antidote – a substance or drug that neutralizes a poison or opposes the effect of a poison.

Antiemetic – a substance or drug that prevents and/or treats nausea and vomiting.

Antiepileptic – a substance or drug that prevents and/or treats epilepsy or seizures. Often used synonymously with the term "anticonvulsant."

Antifungal – a substance or drug that kills and/or prevents the reproduction of fungi.

Antihistamine – prevents the release or blocks the action of histamine, a mediator of allergic reactions, stomach acid production, and mental alertness/wakefulness.

Antiplatelet – a substance or drug that opposes the activity of platelets. Platelets play a major role in blood clot formation.

Antipsychotic – a substance or drug that prevents and/or treats psychosis (e.g. bipolar disorder, schizophrenia).

Antipyretic – a substance or drug that reduces fever.

Antitussive – a substance or drug that suppresses a cough.

Antiviral – a substance or drug that treats viral infections.

Arteries – blood vessels that carry oxygenated blood from the heart to the organs.

Atherosclerosis – hardening and occlusion of arteries caused by the build-up of calcium and cholesterol.

Atrial Fibrillation – a type of cardiac arrhythmia in which a specific area of the heart (the right atrium) receives irregular electrical impulses from the nervous system, causing a rapid, irregular heartbeat. This irregular heartbeat can cause blood clots capable of traveling to the brain and causing strokes. Abbreviations for atrial fibrillation include "AF" and "A-fib."

Benign Prostatic Hyperplasia (BPH) – non-cancerous growth/enlargement of the prostate gland. The enlarged prostate presses against the urethra, blocking the outflow of urine.

Blood Glucose – a measure of the concentration of glucose (sugar) in the blood. High blood glucose (see "hyperglycemia") is a sign of diabetes.

Blood Clot – a mass of coagulated blood capable of blocking blood flow.

Bradycardia – below normal heart rate. (Normal resting heart rate is 60-90 beats per minute.)

Cardiac Arrhythmia – any condition in which the heart beats irregularly (e.g. beats off rhythm, beats too fast, beats too slow).

Cardiovascular System – an organ system composed of the heart and the blood vessels (arteries and veins).

Ceiling Effect – a phenomenon where the therapeutic effect increases only up to a certain point (the "ceiling"). Higher doses impart no additional benefit, causing additional side effects without increasing the therapeutic effect.

Cholesterol – a fatty substance the body uses to produce hormones and cell walls. Excess cholesterol accumulates in arterial blood vessels, causing atherosclerosis and increasing the risk of heart attack.

Cholinergic – a substance or drug that produces or mimics the effects of acetylcholine.

Chronic – a symptom or condition that worsens slowly over time, sometimes progressing undetected. The opposite of acute.

Clean Room – a controlled area designated for sterile compounding. Another term for clean room is "buffer area." The air quality in a clean room should be at least ISO class 7.

Contraceptive – a drug or device that prevents conception/pregnancy.

Coronary Artery Disease (CAD) – narrowing of the arteries that supply blood to the heart, typically caused by atherosclerosis.

Corticosteroid – an anti-inflammatory drug that mimics the hormone "cortisol" which is produced by the adrenal gland. Examples include hydrocortisone and prednisone.

Decongestant – a substance or drug that reduces nasal congestion.

Depressant – a substance or drug that decreases nerve activity, potentially to the point of sedation.

Diuresis – increased urine production. Diuretic drugs (loop diuretics, thiazide diuretics, and potassium-sparing diuretics) work by inducing diuresis.

Edema – swelling. Treatment for edema usually involves a loop diuretic.

Electrolytes – electrically charged minerals. Examples include potassium, calcium, and sodium. Electrolytes are essential for normal body function (e.g. muscle contraction and nerve function).

Elimination – the excretion of a waste product from the body. In many cases, the liver metabolizes and deactivates a drug and then the kidneys transfer the waste product into the urine for elimination.

Embolism – obstruction of a blood vessel by some form of debris or foreign body; for example, a blood clot, a mass of cholesterol, or an air bubble.

Emesis – vomiting.

Enzyme – a catalyst for a chemical reaction. The body naturally produces certain enzymes.

Epistaxis – nosebleed.

Expectorant – a substance or drug that thins mucus, making it easier to expel/cough up.

Glaucoma – a disease characterized by increased intraocular pressure.

Gout – a disease characterized by severe joint pain and inflammation.

Heart Failure – a condition in which the heart is unable to pump forcefully or effectively enough to meet the needs of the body.

Hepatic – pertaining to the liver.

High Efficiency Particulate Air (HEPA) Filter – an special air filter that removes 99.97% of particles that are 0.3 microns (0.00003 centimeters) in diameter or larger.

Histamine – a substance produced within the body that, when released, elicits symptoms associated with allergic reactions, such as runny nose, itchy/watery eyes, and rashes. Histamine also plays a role in stomach acid production and mental alertness/wakefulness.

HMG-CoA Reductase – the key enzyme involved in hepatic cholesterol production.

Hormone – a substance produced by the body to regulate or stimulate certain physiologic functions. Examples of hormones include insulin, estrogen, progesterone, and testosterone.

Hyperglycemia – abnormally high level of glucose in the blood.

Hyperkalemia – abnormally high level of potassium in the blood.

Hypertension – high blood pressure.

Hyperuricemia – abnormally high uric acid levels in the blood.

Hypoglycemia – abnormally low level of glucose in the blood.

Hypokalemia – abnormally low level of potassium in the blood.

Hypotension – low blood pressure.

Indication – a use for a drug; a condition or symptom for which a drug is effective in treating. For example, hypertension is an indication for Lisinopril. In other words, Lisinopril is effective in treating high blood pressure.

ISO Classification – an air quality rating. ISO stand for the "International Organization for Standardization."

Lacrimation – the production of tears.

Laminar Airflow Hood (LAFH) – a combined air filtration machine and workbench. The LAFH collects air from its surrounding environment, usually a clean room, passes it through two filters (a standard filter and a HEPA filter), and then propels the filtered air across the workbench to create an ultra-low particle environment ideal for sterile compounding.

Lipids – fats.

Metabolism – the body's natural process of chemically altering or breaking down a substance (e.g. a drug) with the goal of removing the substance from the body.

Myocardial Infarction (MI) – an event in which a portion of heart muscle tissue dies due to occlusion of the coronary artery.

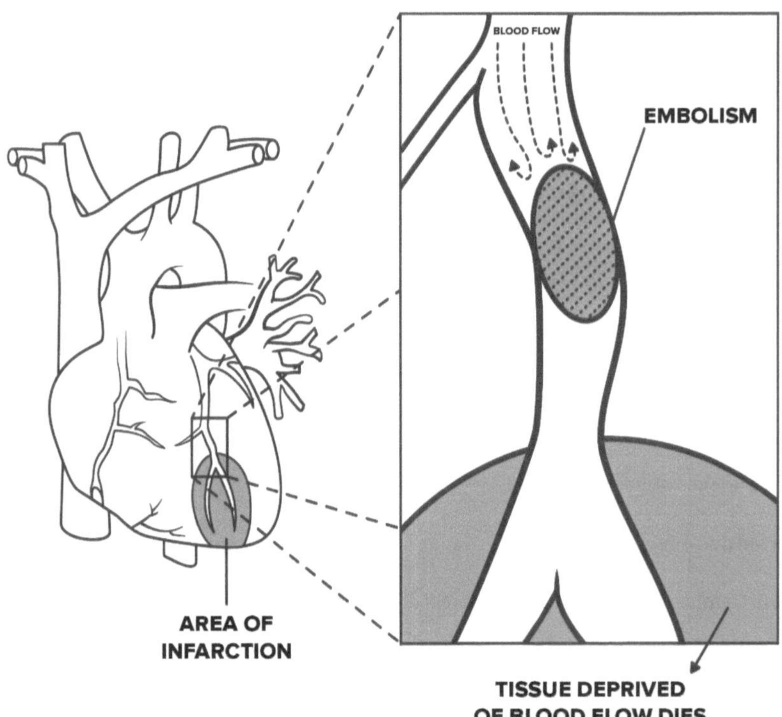

Nephron – the most basic unit of the kidney. Diuretic drugs work by modulating electrolyte exchange at certain locations in the nephron; for example, loop diuretics prevent sodium from being re-absorbed from the Loop of Henle (a segment of the nephron).

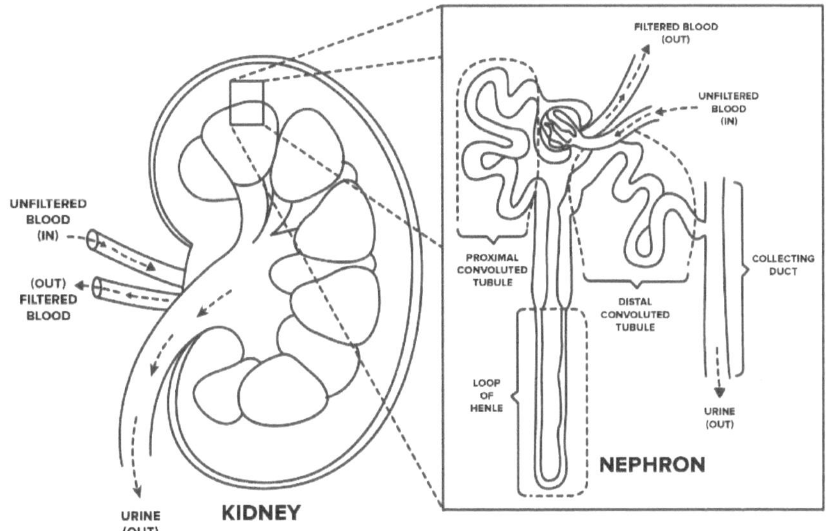

Neuron – a nerve cell; the most basic unit of the nervous system.

Neurotransmitter – a substance released by neurons to manage nervous system-mediated functions. One example is serotonin, which helps manage behavior and mood.

Nitric Oxide – a chemical in the body that causes blood vessels to dilate/expand.

Nonproductive Cough – dry cough.

Non-Steroidal Anti-Inflammatory Drugs (NSAIDs) – medications that work similar to corticosteroids, reducing pain and swelling caused by inflammation.

Off-Label – a term that describes uses for a drug that are not FDA-approved.

Osmosis – the process by which water naturally crosses a semipermeable membrane from the side with low solute concentration to the side with high solute concentration in an attempt to equalize the solute concentration on each side of the membrane.

Peripheral Neuropathy – tingling and/or pain in the extremities caused by nerve damage.

Phosphodiesterase-5 (PDE-5) – a key enzyme involved in the breakdown of nitric oxide.

Photosensitivity – increased sensitivity to sunlight, resulting in a predisposition to sunburn.

Polyuria – excessive urine production.

Pregnancy Category – a rating that summarizes the risk of using of a particular drug during pregnancy. The pregnancy categories are A, B, C, D, and X, where "A" is the least likely to cause birth defects and "X" is the most likely to cause birth defects. Pregnant women should never use a drug with a pregnancy category X rating. The use of a pregnancy category A, B, C, or D drug during pregnancy may be appropriate if the benefits outweigh the risks.

Priapism – a painful, prolonged erection.

Prophylaxis – a measure or action taken to prevent disease. Synonymous with "prevention."

Prostaglandins – a group of chemicals naturally produced and released within the body for various functions, including the promotion of inflammation.

QT Interval – the time between the Q-wave and T-wave on an electrocardiogram. Some drugs can prolong the QT interval, potentially causing life threatening cardiac arrhythmias.

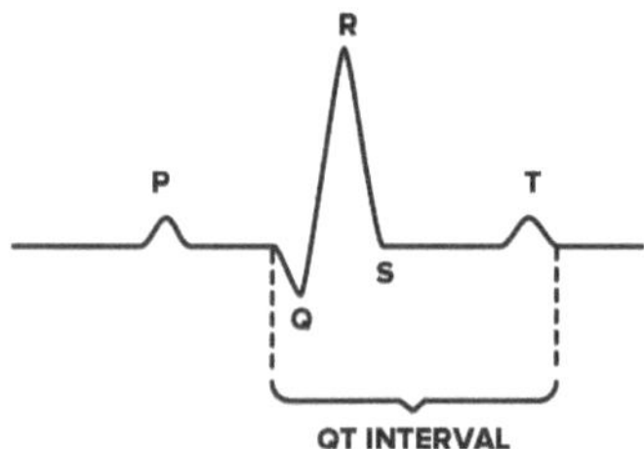

Renal – pertaining to the kidney (e.g. "renal failure" and "kidney failure" are synonymous). The kidneys function as a filtration system for blood.

Sedative-Hypnotic – a substance or drug that induces sleep. Also referred to as tranquilizer.

Serotonin Syndrome – a condition caused by excessive stimulation of serotonin receptors.

Side Effects – the undesired effects/consequences of medication use.

Solute – a substance or drug that is dissolved in a solution.

Solution – the liquid that contains a dissolved substance or drug; a homogeneous mixture composed of a solute and a solvent.

Solvent – the liquid part of a solution in which the solute is dissolved.

Stevens-Johnson syndrome (SJS) – a disease characterized by fever and severe skin rashes involving the mouth, eyes, and mucous membranes.

Stimulant – a substance or drug that increases nerve activity.

Stroke – an event in which an area of the brain dies due to insufficient blood flow.
Sulfa Allergy – an allergy to the class of antibiotics known as the sulfonamides.

Symptom – a sign that indicates the presence of a medical condition, disease, or disorder. For example, a sore throat, nasal congestion, mild fever, sneezing and cough are all symptoms of the common cold.

Syncope – pass out; faint.

Tachycardia – abnormally rapid resting heart rate. (Normal resting heart rate is 60-90 beats per minute)

Tolerance – decreased sensitivity to a drug; the acquired capacity to endure large doses with minimal effects.

Vasoconstrictor – a substance or drug that causes contraction/narrowing of a blood vessel, decreasing the volume of blood flowing through the vessel and increasing blood pressure.

Vasodilator – a substance or drug that causes expansion/relaxation of a blood vessel, which increases the volume of blood flowing through the vessel and decreases blood pressure.

Veins – blood vessels that carry deoxygenated blood from the organs back to the heart.

Withdrawal – response to discontinuation of a drug to which a person has become physically or psychologically dependent.

Now that we have reviewed important terms, we are ready to move on to the specific topics outlined on the ExCPT exam blueprint. We will try to fill in any other gaps in knowledge you may have as we go along. So, let's start with "Regulations & Technician Duties."

REGULATIONS & TECHNICIAN DUTIES

THE PHARMACY TECHNICIAN'S ROLE & FUNCTION

What major activities fall under the scope of pharmacy practice?

- Interpreting, evaluating, and implementing prescriptions and medication orders.
- Compounding and dispensing prescriptions.
- Participating in the selection and administration of drugs and medical devices.
- Performing drug utilization reviews and evaluating the appropriateness and safety of new and existing drug therapies.
- Creating and maintaining patient medication profiles and pharmacy records.
- Counseling and advising patients and other healthcare professionals.
- Administering vaccinations and immunizations.
- Performing drug-related research.

Only a licensed pharmacist can perform certain functions, particularly those involving professional judgment. What are some examples?

- Evaluating prescriptions for conformance with legal requirements, authenticity, accuracy, and drug interactions.
- Making determinations of therapeutic equivalency.
- Performing drug utilization reviews and evaluating appropriateness and safety of drug therapy.
- Verifying and checking the work of pharmacy technicians.
- Signing or initialing a record of dispensing.
- Counseling and advising patients.
- Administering vaccinations and immunizations.

What is the pharmacy technician's primary role?

To assist the pharmacist by completing technical tasks that do not require professional judgment.

Pharmacy technicians complete technical tasks that do not require professional judgment. What are some examples?

- Creating and maintaining patient profiles and pharmacy records.
- Receiving written, faxed, and electronically transmitted prescriptions.
- Typing prescription labels.
- Filling prescription orders.
    - Retrieving drugs from stock.
    - Counting or measuring dosage units.
    - Placing dosage units in a container.
    - Affixing a label to the container.
    - Returning drugs to stock.
- Handling or delivering completed prescriptions.
- Alerting the pharmacist to situations that require professional judgment.
- Assisting the pharmacist in managing inventory (e.g. medications, vials/bottles, caps).
- Restocking inventory/placing new items on the shelves.
- Identifying and removing expired products from the inventory.
- Disposing of expired or contaminated products according to policies & procedures.
- Removing and returning recalled, discontinued, and over-stocked items from the pharmacy's inventory.
- Maintaining the organization and cleanliness of the pharmacy and patient care areas.
- Maintaining security of the prescription area.
    - Following procedures intended to prevent unauthorized individuals from entering the pharmacy (e.g. lock the doors, engage the security gate, and activate the alarm during the pharmacist's absence).
- Complying with rules and regulations related to the practice of pharmacy.

Note: all work completed by a pharmacy technician must be checked by a pharmacist.

PRESCRIPTION DEPARTMENT LAYOUT & WORKFLOW

RETAIL AND OTHER OUTPATIENT PHARMACY SETTINGS

Retail pharmacies are typically setup with four distinct technician work areas – prescription drop-off/input, filling, bagging, and prescription pick-up. The technician working at the prescription drop off/input area also helps the pharmacist troubleshoot rejected insurance claims and fix prescriptions that have problems such as missing quantity, invalid DEA or NPI number, etc. In busy pharmacies that employ multiple technicians, the technicians typically take turns rotating through each work area. In slower pharmacies, one technician may cover multiple work areas, switching back and forth as needed. Aside from performing the functions associated with their work area, all technicians are responsible for answering the telephone and responding to customer service requests. In any case, each pharmacy has individualized policies and procedures that dictate workflow.

RETAIL/OUTPATIENT PHARMACY – GENERAL WORKFLOW

- Patient brings one or more new prescriptions and/or refill requests to drop-off area
    - Refills may be requested by telephone
    - New prescriptions may be called, faxed or electronically transmitted to the pharmacy by the prescriber's office
- Technician accepts the prescription(s) & verifies the patient's name and date of birth
    - Ensure this information appears on the face of each new prescription
    - Include patient's address for controlled substance prescriptions
- For returning customers, ask for their prescription drug insurance card, a list of known allergies, and any medical changes if different from last visit
- For new customers, create a new patient profile that includes name, address, telephone number, date of birth, gender, known allergies, medical conditions, current medications (including OTC and herbal) and prescription drug insurance information
- Technician estimates a wait time
    - For example, "Your prescription should be ready in 30 minutes."
- Technician enters ("inputs") the prescription information into the computer
- Pharmacist checks the information entered by the technician to ensure accuracy and to screen for potential drug interactions and contraindications
- Claim is processed electronically through the patient's insurance using the information from the patient's profile (if applicable)
- If claim is rejected, the technician and/or pharmacist explore options for obtaining a paid claim
- Prescriptions for paid claims and self-pay customers enter the filling queue
- Technician fills prescription from the filling queue
- Pharmacist physically checks the filled prescription to verify accuracy
- Pharmacist or technician places verified prescription in a bag with drug information paperwork and a patient identification tag
- Technician transports the completed prescription to the pick-up area
- Technician or cashier processes the financial transaction when the patient arrives

ATTENTION: If at any point during this process the technician notices a potential dispensing error, it is crucial that the technician communicate this information to the pharmacist. Dispensing errors can be fatal.

Note: When contacting a prescriber's office to clarify any part of a prescription, it is important to document the following information on the prescription hardcopy:

1. The details that were verified or changed.
2. The name of the person with whom you spoke.
3. The date and time of the conversation.
4. Your name or initials.

INSTITUTIONAL AND OTHER INPATIENT PHARMACY SETTINGS

Institutional pharmacies, such as a pharmacy department that serves inpatients in a hospital, are typically setup with two distinct technician work areas – the order processing area and the clean room. The order processing area is where prepackaged medications are stored. The clean room is where the preparation of sterile infusions takes place. In large institutional pharmacies that employ several technicians, each technician usually works in one area for their entire shift, rotating between areas on a daily or weekly basis. It is more common in smaller institutional pharmacies for the technicians to switch back and forth between work areas throughout the day as necessary.

INSTITUTIONAL/INPATIENT PHARMACY – GENERAL WORKFLOW

CART FILL FOR DAILY DOSES*

- Technician or pharmacist prints list of active medication orders for each inpatient
- Technician retrieves medications detailed on the list for each patient, placing the medications in the patient's assigned compartment in the medication cart
- Pharmacist checks each compartment of the cart to ensure that patients receive the correct medications and doses
- Technician delivers medication cart to the wards
- This process occurs once at the beginning of each day

FILLING NEW DAILY ORDERS AND ONE-TIME DOSES

- Prescriber submits a new medication order
- Pharmacist checks medication order and screens for potential drug interactions and contraindications
- Pharmacist prints label for the medication order
- Technician fills the medication order according to the details on the label**
- Pharmacist checks the medication order filled by the technician to ensure accuracy
- Stat orders are delivered to the wards immediately by the technician
- Non-urgent orders accumulate and are delivered to the wards periodically by the technician based on a delivery schedule (e.g. every 2 hours)

Note: Pharmacists typically fill controlled substance orders and a pharmacy technician delivers the orders to the wards. It is standard procedure in inpatient facilities for a nurse to witness and sign for the delivery of any controlled substance medications.

*Most patients have medication orders that nurses administer on a scheduled basis for several days in a row, such as blood pressure medications or IV antibiotic infusions. Technicians fill these orders during a once daily routine called "cart fill." The cart used in a cart fill contains a separate compartment for each patient, and technicians fill the cart with each patient's scheduled doses for that day and deliver the cart to the patient floor (wards) once every morning.

**Some medication orders are for sterile infusions that require admixture by a technician in the clean room. Technicians working in the order processing area fill orders for prepackaged and non-sterile items (e.g. tablets, capsules, oral solutions, and prepackaged injections).

BASIC INVENTORY MANAGEMENT

Managing the inventory in a pharmacy is straightforward. When supplies are low, order more. When a patient needs a drug that is not in stock, order the drug. When an item is expired or recalled, remove it from the shelf and dispose or return the product according to the pharmacy's policies and procedures. Despite the simplicity, there are three concepts that we are going to dissect in this section. 1) Maintaining par levels to ensure there is enough medication on-hand to meet the normal demands of the customers, 2) rotating stock to reduce the likelihood that the pharmacy will dispense new inventory before older inventory, and 3) removing expired and recalled products from stock.

MAINTAINING PAR LEVELS

The par level is the minimum quantity of a drug (or other product) that must be on-hand for the business to meet day-to-day customer needs. For instance, if a pharmacy dispenses 600 tablets of Lisinopril 20 mg tablets on average each day, then the par level for that drug should be set somewhere around 2,000 tablets. This will ensure the pharmacy has enough medication on-hand to cover a full business day plus weekends when there are no deliveries. When the inventory of a drug or product falls below the par level, the pharmacy must place an order to replenish the inventory. Most pharmacies have an automated inventory replenishment system. In these cases, the pharmacy computer is programmed to place a replenishment order automatically when the inventory drops below par level recorded in the computerized inventory record. For this process to work, it is crucial that inventory records are accurate and up-to-date.

ROTATING STOCK

When a pharmacy receives a shipment of medications from a distributor or manufacturer, the pharmacy technician places each medication in its assigned location on the shelf (usually in alphabetical order). When placing newly received items on the shelf, it is important to rotate the stock. In other words, move the older items toward the front edge of the shelf and place the new items behind the older items. This helps ensure that the pharmacy dispenses the older medications sooner, thus reducing the chance of accumulating expired medications. Expired medications are ineffective, potentially unsafe, and cannot be dispensed.

REMOVING EXPIRED & RECALLED PRODUCTS FROM STOCK

On a periodic basis (e.g. monthly), pharmacy personnel must check the items in the pharmacy's inventory to ensure that any expired products are removed from stock. Pharmacies also receive notification of recalls from manufacturers whenever they occur. Pharmacy personnel must respond quickly to recall notifications by removing recalled items from stock. Expired and recalled products must be removed promptly to prevent patients from receiving unsafe and ineffective products.

LOT NUMBERS & EXPIRATION DATES

Are all drug products required to possess a lot number?
Yes, all drug products must have a lot number displayed on the package label.

What are lot numbers and why are they important?
The lot number is a unique identifier consisting of a series of numbers and/or letters as assigned by the manufacturer. Manufacturers produce drug products in large batches, and the lot number identifies the batch from which the contents of that container originated. Lot numbers play a crucial role in recalls. If a manufacturer distributes a drug product to pharmacies and subsequently discovers an abnormality, such as discoloration or contamination, then they will recall the affected batch. Pharmacies use the lot number to identify and remove the recalled product from their inventory, thus preventing distribution to patients.

What happens if a drug product has no lot number (e.g. the label was torn or scuffed and the lot number is no longer visible)?
Containers of a recalled drug that are missing their lot number must be treated the same as a recalled container.

Are all prescription drugs required to have an expiration date?
Yes, the FDA requires manufacturers to assign expiration dates for all prescription drugs.

Is it acceptable to use or dispense a drug product that is expired?
No. The expiration date is the final date through which the manufacturer can guarantee the potency and safety of the drug.

If a drug product has an expiration date of 08/2018. Will the product be "expired" on 08/02/2018?
No, the drug will be expired on the final day of 08/2018, which would be 08/31/2018.

What is unique about the expiration date for a vial of insulin?
A vial of insulin can be used for 28 days after the rubber stopper has been punctured or up until the expiration date printed on the vial, whichever comes first.

The date is July 14, 2016. You are working as a pharmacy technician in a hospital and a nurse asks you, "When do I have to dispose of this vial of insulin?" The expiration date printed on the vial reads "EXP: 09/31/2016," but the nurse informs you that she initially opened the vial on July 1, 2016. What is the final day this vial of insulin can be used?

A. 07/14/2016
B. 07/29/2016
C. 07/30/2016
D. 09/31/2016

Answer:
Since insulin comes in a multi-dose vial, we must assign a beyond-use date equal to 28 days from the date of first use. For that reason, choice "B" is correct.

B. 07/29/2016

FDA RECALLS

Class I Recalls
Use of (or exposure to) the recalled product will cause serious adverse health consequences up to and including death.

Class II Recalls
Use of (or exposure to) the recalled product could cause temporary or medically reversible adverse health consequences.

Class III Recalls
Use of the recalled product is unlikely to cause adverse health consequences.

REVIEW QUESTION:
What is the most serious class of FDA recall?
Class I recall.

CONTROLLED SUBSTANCE SCHEDULES

Schedule I Controlled Substances

Examples: GHB, heroin

- No accepted medical use.
- Not legal for prescribing purposes.
- High potential for abuse.
- Lack safety.

Schedule II Controlled Substances

Examples: MS Contin® (morphine sulfate ER), Roxicodone® (oxycodone)

- Accepted medical use.
- Available by prescription only.
- High potential for abuse.
- High potential for physical/psychological dependence.

Schedule III Controlled Substances

Examples: AndroGel® (testosterone), Marinol® (dronabinol), Subutex® (buprenorphine)

- Accepted medical use.
- Available by prescription only.
- Moderate potential for abuse.
- Moderate-low potential for physical/psychological dependence.

Schedule IV Controlled Substances

Examples: Valium® (diazepam), Xanax® (alprazolam), Provigil® (modafinil)

- Accepted medical use.
- Available by prescription only.
- Mild potential for abuse.
- Mild potential for physical/psychological dependence.

Schedule V Controlled Substances

Examples: Lomotil® (diphenoxylate/atropine), Cheratussin® AC (guaifenesin/codeine)

- Accepted medical use.
- Available by prescription; limited quantities available OTC in some states.
- Low potential for abuse.
- Low potential for physical/psychological dependence.

COMMON CONTROLLED SUBSTANCES CATEGORIZED BY SCHEDULE

It is important to recognize the schedule to which a controlled substance belongs. See below for our list of the most recognized and prescribed controlled substances categorized by schedule. Note: Some students will realize that the laws in their state result in stricter scheduling of certain controlled substances, but keep in mind that the ExCPT will test your knowledge of federal laws and regulations, not state laws and regulations. The information below was derived from the federal Controlled Substances Act (CSA). Generic names are listed with brand names in parenthesis.

Schedule I Controlled Substances

- GHB
- Heroin
- LSD
- Marijuana (**Note:** used medically in some states, but not legal for medical use according to *federal* law)
- MDMA

Schedule II Controlled Substances

C-II Opioids:

- codeine
- hydrocodone*
- morphine (MS Contin®, Kadian®, Roxanol®)
- meperidine (Demerol®)
- methadone (Dolophine®, Methadose®)
- fentanyl (Duragesic®)
- hydromorphone (Dilaudid®, Exalgo®)
- oxycodone (Roxicodone®, Oxycontin®)
- oxymorphone (Opana®)

*Effective October 6, 2014, this includes all hydrocodone combination products (e.g. Norco®, Lortab®, Vicodin®, Vicoprofen®, Tussionex®).

C-II Stimulants:

- amphetamine/dextroamphetamine (Adderall®)
- cocaine
- methamphetamine (Desoxyn®)
- methylphenidate (Concerta®, Metadate®, Methylin®, Ritalin®)

C-II Depressants:

- amobarbital (Amytal®)
- pentobarbital (Nembutal®)
- secobarbital (Seconal®)

C-II Hallucinogens:

- nabilone (Cesamet®)

Schedule III Controlled Substances

C-III Opioids:

- buprenorphine (Buprenex®, Subutex®)
- buprenorphine/naloxone (Suboxone®)
- camphorated tincture of opium (Paregoric®)
- codeine* (e.g. Tylenol #3, Fioricet with codeine)

*Categorized as a C-III controlled when used in limited quantities *in combination with other medications*.

C-III Mixed Opioid Agonist/Antagonists:

- nalorphine (Nalline®)

C-III Stimulants:

- benzphetamine (Didrex®, Regimex)
- phendimetrazine (Bontril®)

C-III Depressants:

- barbituric acid and its derivatives
- ketamine (Ketalar®)

The following Schedule II depressants are considered Schedule III when they exist in a compound, mixture, or suppository form:

- amobarbital
- pentobarbital
- secobarbital

C-III Anabolic Steroids:

All anabolic steroids are C-III according to federal law.

- testosterone (AndroGel®, Testim®, Axiron®, Depo-Testosterone®)
- oxandrolone (Oxandrin®)

C-III Hallucinogens:

- dronabinol (Marinol®)

Schedule IV Controlled Substances

C-IV Depressants (Benzodiazepines):

All prescription benzodiazepines are federally classified as Schedule IV. The best way to recognize a benzodiazepine is by the last part of its generic name. The generic name usually ends in "–azepam" or "–azolam."

- alprazolam (Xanax®)
- chlordiazepoxide (Librium®)
  - The first benzodiazepine formally discovered
  - The only benzodiazepine whose generic name ends in "–epoxide."
- clonazepam (Klonopin®)
- clorazepate (Tranxene®)
  - One of only two benzodiazepines whose generic name ends in "–ate."
- diazepam (Valium®, Diastat®)
- estazolam (Prosom®)
- flurazepam (Dalmane®)
- lorazepam (Ativan®)
- midazolam (Versed®)
- temazepam (Restoril®)

C-IV Depressants:

- eszopiclone (Lunesta®)
- zaleplon (Sonata®)
- zolpidem (Ambien®)
- phenobarbital (Luminal®)
- carisoprodol (Soma®)
- tramadol (Ultram®)

C-IV Mixed Opioid Agonist/Antagonists:

- butorphanol (Stadol®)
- pentazocine (Talwin®)

C-IV Stimulants:

- modafinil (Provigil®)
- phentermine (Adipex-P®, Suprenza®)
- phentermine/topiramate (Qsymia®)
- sibutramine (Meridia®)

Schedule V Controlled Substances

C-V Opioids:

- codeine with guaifenesin (Robitussin® AC)
- diphenoxylate with atropine (Lomotil®)

C-V Depressants:

- pregabalin (Lyrica®)
- lacosamide (Vimpat®)

For the complete list of controlled substances, go to:
<http://www.deadiversion.usdoj.gov/schedules/orangebook/e_cs_sched.pdf>

CONTROLLED SUBSTANCE LAWS

True or false. Pharmacies can dispense Schedule I controlled substances pursuant to a valid, hand-signed prescription.
False, Schedule I controlled substances are not legal for medical use.

In what setting might you find Schedule I controlled substances?
The only setting in which a Schedule I controlled substance can be legally utilized is a research laboratory registered with the DEA.

True or false. Schedule II controlled substance prescription records can be stored in the same file as other prescription medications.
False, Schedule II prescription records must be stored separate from all other prescription records.

After an initial inventory of controlled substances has been taken, such as when a new pharmacy first opens for business, how frequently must an inventory of controlled substances be conducted?
At least once every two years.

According to the federal Controlled Substances Act (CSA), how should you store Schedule III – V prescription files?
Either separately from all other prescription records or in such a way that they are readily retrievable from the non-controlled prescription records (e.g. Schedule III – V prescription records can be stored along with non-controlled substance prescription records if each controlled substance prescription is marked with the letter "C" in red ink).

When Schedule II controlled substances are sent to a reverse distributor because they are expired, damaged, or otherwise unusable, what form should be used?
DEA Form 222.

Who would be responsible for filling out the Form 222?
The reverse distributor – the entity receiving the substance is always the one that fills out the form.

When Schedule III – V controlled substances are returned, is a DEA Form 222 necessary?
No, Schedule III – V controlled substances may be transferred via invoice (DEA Form 222 is only used for Schedule I and II controlled substances).

How long must the pharmacy keep controlled substance return records, prescription records, and inventory records?
2 years.

What information must be included on a controlled substance prescription?

1. Patient's full name
2. Patient's address
3. Prescriber's full name
4. Prescribers work address
5. Prescriber's DEA number
6. Drug name
7. Drug strength
8. Dosage form
9. Quantity prescribed
10. Directions for use
11. Number of refills authorized (if any)

True or false. Federal law prohibits e-prescribing of C-II drugs.
False, federal law permits e-prescribing of C-II through C-V drugs; however, the software used by the prescriber sending the prescription and the pharmacy receiving the prescription must be certified by the DEA.

According to federal law, C-II prescriptions must be filled within how many days after being signed by the prescriber?
Federal law places no time limit within which a C-II prescription must be filled (i.e. the prescription is considered legally valid for an unlimited period of time after it is issued). Note, however, that individual state laws may impose a time limit.

True or false. For controlled substance prescriptions, the maximum quantity that can be dispensed according to federal law is a 30-day supply.
False, although some states and some insurance companies may limit controlled substance quantities to a 30-day supply, there are no specific federal limits.

Note: When federal and state laws differ, you must follow the more stringent law.

Are verbal orders (i.e. prescriptions that are called in by the prescriber where there is no prescriber-signed prescription hard copy) for C-II prescriptions permitted?
Only in emergencies (as determined by the pharmacist).

Note: The pharmacist must immediately reduce the verbal order to writing and the quantity of medication must be limited to an amount adequate to treat the patient only for the duration of the emergency period.

After calling in an emergency C-II prescription, what must the prescriber do next?
Provide the pharmacy with a written and signed hard copy, which the pharmacy files along with the verbal order.

When emergency C-II prescriptions are called in, a prescriber has how many days to furnish the pharmacy with a written and signed prescription hardcopy?
7 days according to federal law.

True or false. C-II prescriptions may be refilled up to 5 times in 6 months.
False, C-II prescription refills are legally prohibited.

Are C-II prescriptions valid when received by facsimile (fax machine)?

A pharmacy can use a faxed copy of a C-II prescription to fill a prescription; but prior to dispensing, the patient must present the original signed prescription.

What are the three types of prescription orders for which a pharmacy can dispense a faxed C-II prescription without requiring presentation of the original signed prescription?

1. Home infusion orders
2. Long-term care facility orders
3. Hospice care program orders

A patient presents six (6) prescriptions for Adderall 5 mg. Each prescription is written for 30 tablets with the instructions to take 1 tablet by mouth every morning and 1 tablet by mouth every afternoon at 3 PM. Is it legal for the patient to possess this many prescriptions for a C-II drug?

While it would be prudent to verify the prescriptions with the prescriber before dispensing, federal law does permit prescribers to issue multiple C-II prescriptions at one time *as long as the total days' supply does not exceed 90 days.*

Note: these prescriptions would need to have the earliest fill date written on them (e.g. "do not fill until 4/15," "do not fill until 4/30," etc.).

By what means can a prescriber issue C-III, C-IV, and C-V prescriptions?

- Orally/verbally.
- In writing.
- By facsimile (fax).
- Electronically (e-prescribing) where state law permits.

Does the law allow for C-III, C-IV, and C-V prescription refills?

Yes, a prescriber can issue up to five (5) refills for C-III and C-IV prescriptions, but the original prescription and any refills must be filled within six (6) months of the date written. Refill limitations do not apply to C-V prescriptions.

For non-controlled substance prescriptions, a prescriber's agent (e.g. nurse or secretary) may call in a verbal prescription. Can a prescriber's agent call in Schedule III – V prescriptions?

No, the individual prescriber must personally make the call to submit a C-III through V prescription verbally.

Are prescribers required to personally send faxes when C-III – V prescriptions are transmitted to pharmacies by fax?

No, a prescriber's agent may send faxes for C-III, C-IV, and C-V prescriptions.

Can a prescriber post-date a prescription for a controlled substance (e.g. record the date written as 8/14/16 when he/she actually wrote the prescription on 8/12/16)?

No. The prescriber might try to do this when he/she doesn't want the patient to have the prescription filled until 8/14/16, but they should record the written date as 8/12/16 and write on the face of the prescription "do not fill until 8/14/16."

Can a controlled substance be delivered or shipped to an individual in another country if they have a valid prescription?
No, the federal Controlled Substances Act prohibits exportation of controlled substances.

Prescribers that want to prescribe Schedule III – V controlled substances for treatment of narcotic addiction (i.e. products containing buprenorphine) must display what unique identifier on the face of the prescription?
Their unique DEA registration number that begins with the letter "X" must be displayed, which is granted to prescribers that have obtained a special waiver* from the DEA (in addition to their standard DEA registration number).

*Typically, controlled substances used to treat narcotic addiction can only be prescribed, administered, and/or dispensed within a Narcotic Treatment Facility (NTF), but the DEA grants waivers to certain prescribers, allowing them to prescribe, administer, and/or dispense C-III – V prescriptions for treatment of narcotic addiction outside of a NTF.

What must the pharmacy do in the event of theft or loss of a controlled substance?
The pharmacy must notify the DEA and complete a DEA Form 106 to document the details of the theft or loss.

SUMMARY OF FEDERAL CONTROLLED SUBSTANCES ACT REQUIREMENTS

	SCHEDULE II	SCHEDULE III & IV	SCHEDULE V
DEA Registration	Required	Required	Required
Receiving Records	DEA Form 222	Invoices	Invoices
Accepted Prescription Formats	Written or Electronic	Written, Verbal, Faxed, or Electronic	Written, Verbal, Faxed, Electronic or OTC*
Refills	No	No more than 5 within 6 months	As authorized when prescription is issued
Distribution Between Registrants	DEA Form 222	Invoices	Invoices
Theft or Significant Loss	Report and complete DEA Form 106	Report and complete DEA Form 106	Report and complete DEA Form 106

Note: Keep all controlled substance records for two (2) years.
Exceptions: Faxed C-II prescriptions are valid for home infusion, long-term care, and hospice patients. Verbal C-II prescriptions are valid in emergencies, as long as the prescribing practitioner provides the pharmacy with a signed hardcopy within seven (7) days.
* Where authorized by state law.

CONTROLLED SUBSTANCE REFILLS

C-II:	Refills not permitted
C-III & C-IV:	Refills permitted, up to 5 refills valid for 6 months
C-V:	Refills permitted, no maximum

CONTROLLED SUBSTANCE PARTIAL FILLS

C-II:	Partial fills permitted if the remainder can be filled within 72 hours.*
C-III, C-IV, & C-V:	Partial fills permitted with no time limit for filling the remainder.

*Most C-II medication orders take longer than 3 days to arrive, so most pharmacists refuse to partial fill schedule II controlled substance prescriptions.

CONTROLLED SUBSTANCE PRESCRIPTION RECORDS

C-II:	Must keep separate from all other prescriptions.
C-III, C-IV, & C-V:	Keep separate from all other prescriptions, or mark in the lower right corner with the letter "C" at least 1-inch high in red ink and store in the same file with non-controlled substance prescriptions.
Note:	For pharmacies that dispense controlled substance e-prescriptions, the prescription records can be stored electronically as long as they can be sorted by prescriber name, patient name, drug dispensed, and date filled and the records are printable or capable of being transferred to a government or law enforcement agency.

CONTROLLED SUBSTANCE PRESCRIPTION TRANSFERS

C-II:	Not transferable between pharmacies.
C-III, C-IV, & C-V:	Patients can transfer each prescription to another pharmacy one time; however, multiple transfers may take place between pharmacies that share a real-time online database. Licensed pharmacists must complete all controlled substance transfers. Pharmacy technicians cannot transfer controlled substance prescriptions.

CONTROLLED SUBSTANCE STORAGE AND SECURITY

C-II:	Store in a locked cabinet or among the non-controlled medications in such a manner as to obstruct theft or diversion.
C-III, C-IV, & C-V:	Same as for C-II. Store in a locked cabinet or among the non-controlled medications in such a manner as to obstruct theft or diversion.

OVER-THE-COUNTER SCHEDULE V CONTROLLED SUBSTANCE SALES

As mentioned in the table summarizing federal Controlled Substances Act requirements, federal law permits over-the-counter (OTC) selling of schedule V controlled substances. As you know, the term "over-the-counter" means the medication is available directly to the consumer without a prescription; however, since these particular drugs are controlled substances, there are strict quantity limits and recordkeeping requirements.

Quantity Limits for OTC Schedule V Controlled Substances

An individual customer can purchase up to one of the following in a 48-hour period:

- 8 ounces (240 mL) of a liquid controlled substance that contains opium.
- 4 ounces (120 mL) of a liquid that contains a controlled substance other than opium.
- 48 dosage units of a solid controlled substance that contains opium.
- 24 dosage units of a solid that contains a controlled substance other than opium.

Recordkeeping Requirements for OTC Schedule V Controlled Substances

- Require every purchaser to furnish identification.
- Ensure each purchaser is at least 18 years old.
- Record the following details in a record book:
    - Name & address of purchaser.
    - Name & quantity of controlled substance dispensed.*
    - Date of purchase.
    - Name or initials of the dispensing pharmacist.
- The pharmacy must keep records for at least 2 years from the date of last entry, as is the case for all controlled substance records.

*A pharmacist must dispense the controlled substance, but a pharmacy technician can execute the financial transaction.

Note: Some states prohibit the OTC sale of schedule V controlled substances, but the ExCPT tests your knowledge of federal law.

OVER-THE-COUNTER PSEUDOEPHEDRINE SALES

Pseudoephedrine is the active ingredient in Sudafed, a powerful OTC decongestant. It is also an active ingredient in many other allergy, cough and cold products (e.g. Mucinex-D, Zyrtec-D, Advil Cold & Sinus). Pseudoephedrine itself is not a controlled substance, but it is a precursor to the Schedule II controlled substance methamphetamine. Criminals can convert pseudoephedrine into this addictive drug for illegal use or sale, but they need large quantities of pseudoephedrine to do this. For that reason, pseudoephedrine is stored behind the pharmacy counter or in a locked cabinet kept away from customers to prevent theft. Customers are limited to the amount of pseudoephedrine they can purchase on a daily and monthly basis, and the pharmacy must record each sale.

REQUIREMENTS AND LIMITS FOR SELLING OTC PSEUDOEPHEDRINE

- Customer must present a photo ID
- Manufacturers must package pseudoephedrine tablets and capsules in blister packs* (see image to right)

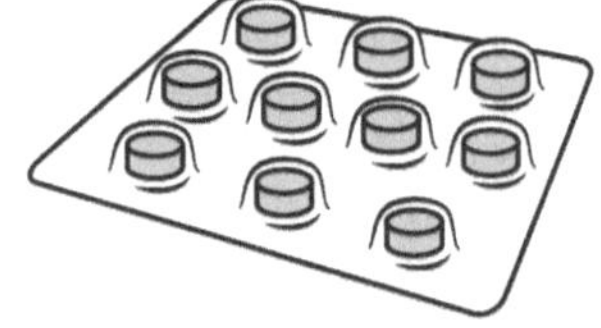

- Individual daily limit is 3.6 grams of pseudoephedrine
- Individual monthly limit is 9 grams*

*The monthly (30-day) purchase limit is 7.5 grams for products purchased via mail order.

- The following information must be recorded from each sale:
    - Product name
    - Quantity
    - Name and address of purchaser
    - Date and time of sale
    - Signature of purchaser
- Records must be kept for at least 2 years

*Removing medication from a blister pack can be difficult. By packaging pseudoephedrine-containing products in blister packs, we are making it harder for criminals to access the large amounts of pseudoephedrine needed to manufacture methamphetamine.

Note: The quantity limits and recordkeeping requirements outlined above do not apply to patients receiving a pseudoephedrine product pursuant to a valid prescription.

SUMMARY OF PSEUDOEPHEDRINE SALES LIMITS (PER CUSTOMER)

24-HOUR LIMIT (RETAIL OR MAIL ORDER)	30-DAY LIMIT (RETAIL)	30-DAY LIMIT (MAIL ORDER)
3.6 grams	9 grams	7.5 grams

DEA FORMS

The Drug Enforcement Administration (DEA) is responsible for enforcing the federal Controlled Substances Act (CSA). The DEA's goal is to ensure that controlled substances are available for legitimate medical and research uses, while preventing illicit use and illegal distribution. To accomplish this, the DEA strictly monitors the manufacturing, distribution, and dispensing of controlled substances. This monitoring requires extensive documentation by entities that handle controlled substances. To standardize recordkeeping procedures, the DEA provides preformatted forms for pharmacies and other businesses that handle controlled substances. See the chart below. Memorize the title of each form (the "DEA Form Number") and its associated purpose/use.

DEA FORM NUMBER	PURPOSE/USE
DEA Form 41	For reporting the destruction of controlled substances.
DEA Form 104	For reporting a pharmacy closure or surrender of a pharmacy permit.
DEA Form 106	For reporting the loss or theft of controlled substances.
DEA Form 222	For ordering Schedule II controlled substances.
DEA Form 222a	For ordering additional DEA 222 Forms.
DEA Form 224	For applying for a DEA registration number.
DEA Form 224a	For renewing DEA registration (renewal is required every 3 years).

Note: Research laboratories also use the DEA Form 222 for ordering Schedule I controlled substances.

For pharmacies, the most commonly used among these is the DEA Form 222. For that reason, you should be very familiar with this particular form and its use. See below for an outline of important details regarding the DEA Form 222:

- Each form includes 2 carbon copies (the original, plus 2 attached copies)
- The first page (original) is brown
  - Must be retained by the drug supplier
- The second page (first carbon copy) is green
  - Must be forwarded to the DEA by the drug supplier
- The third page (second carbon copy) is blue
  - Must be retained by the pharmacy
- Mistakes cannot be corrected
  - When an erroneous entry is made, all copies of the form must be voided and retained by the pharmacy

When ordering Schedule II drugs for your pharmacy, what do you do with the first two pages (brown and green) of the DEA Form 222?
Give them to the supplier without separating them. For the form to be valid from the supplier's perspective, the brown and green copies must be intact with the carbon paper between them. The pharmacy must retain the third page (blue copy) of the form.

Note: Pharmacies are require to keep all controlled substance records, including executed DEA forms, for at least 2 years.

DEA NUMBER VERIFICATION

Sample DEA#: MH4836726

Why and how would you determine if a prescriber's DEA number is legitimate?
A prescriber cannot legally issue a controlled substance prescription unless he/she has obtained a DEA registration number. That number must appear on the face of every controlled substance prescription issued by the prescriber. You may want to verify a DEA number before dispensing a controlled substance, especially if you or the pharmacist suspect forgery. There are two components of a DEA number: the letters and the numbers. First, we will look at the letters.

The 1st Letter: DEA numbers begin with 2 letters. The 1st letter of the DEA number identifies the type of practitioner or registrant.

- A, B, or F for physicians, dentists, veterinarians, hospitals, and pharmacies
- M for midlevel practitioners
- P or R for drug distributors

Note: prescribers with a DEA waiver to write prescriptions for Subutex® or Suboxone® outside of a narcotic treatment facility (NTF) have an additional DEA number that begins with the letter "X."

The 2nd Letter: The second letter of the DEA number will be the same as the first letter of the prescriber's last name or the first letter in the name of the business.

Now that you know what the letters in a DEA number represent, let's see how to go about verifying the numerical portion of a DEA number.

---**Step 1**---

Add the 1st, 3rd, and 5th digits of the DEA number.

---**Step 2**---

Add the 2nd, 4th, and 6th digits of the DEA number and multiply the sum by 2.

Note: Remember to multiply the correct set of numbers by 2. Many students mistakenly multiply the sum of the 1st, 3rd, and 5th digits by 2 and get the wrong answer.

---**Step 3**---

Take your answer from "Step 1" and add it to your answer from "Step 2."

---**Step 4**---

Your answer for "Step 3" will be a 2-digit number. If the DEA number is legitimate, then the second digit of this 2-digit number will match the 7th and final digit of the DEA number. For example, imagine your answer from "Step 3" was 4<u>8</u>. If legitimate, then the DEA number would end with the number 8. Now try it yourself. Use this 4-step process to verify the sample DEA# shown at the top of this page, and then try to do the sample problem on the following page.

PRACTICE PROBLEM

Verify the DEA number shown below.

John Smith, MD
DEA # FS8524616

SOLUTION

- The registrant is a physician (MD), so the first letter must be "A, B, or F."
- The prescriber's last name is Smith, so the second letter must be "S."
- The sum of the 1st, 3rd, and 5th numbers (8 + 2 + 6) is 16.
- The sum of the 2nd, 4th, and 6th numbers (5 + 4 + 1) is 10, and 10 x 2 = 20.
- The sum of 16 and 20 is 3$\underline{6}$.
- The last digit of the DEA number is 6, which is the same as the second digit of the number 36.
- According to our analysis, this DEA number appears to be legitimate.

Note: The "Drug Addiction Treatment Act of 2000" (DATA 2000) is the name of the law that requires prescribers to include their special DEA number (which starts with the letter "X") on prescriptions written for Subutex® or Suboxone®. For example, Dr. John Smith's special DEA number (if he had one) would look like this: XS8524616.

HEALTH INSURANCE PORTABILITY & ACCOUNTABILITY ACT

What is the purpose of the Health Insurance Portability and Accountability Act (HIPAA)?
To protect the privacy of individual health information (referred to in the law as "protected health information" or "PHI").

If an individual's PHI has been breached, what must be done according to HIPAA?
The pharmacy must notify the individual that his/her PHI was exposed. This is known as the "HIPAA Breach Notification Rule."

Does HIPAA set standards for protecting electronic PHI, such as electronic medical records (EMR)?
Yes.

When using or disclosing PHI, what principle should you keep in mind?
The principle of "minimum necessary use and disclosure."

To which situation(s) does the principle of "minimum necessary use and disclosure" not apply?

- Disclosures to a healthcare provider for treatment.
- Disclosures to the patient upon request.
- Disclosures authorized by the patient.
- Disclosures necessary to comply with other laws.
- Disclosures to the Department of Health and Human Services (HHS) for a compliance investigation, review, or enforcement.

What are some practical measures you can take to protect a patient's privacy?

- Maintain a reasonable distance between the patient you are speaking with and other people in the area to prevent others from overhearing sensitive information/PHI.
- Speak loud enough for the patient to hear you, but not loud enough that bystanders will hear.
- Do not shout to a patient when discussing PHI such as medication names, medical conditions, date of birth, address, and other sensitive information.
- Never gossip about a patient and their medical information.
- Do not disclose PHI over the phone unless the person on the phone is entitled to the information and it is for a legitimate purpose.

GENERIC SUBSTITUTION & THE ORANGE BOOK

Prescribers often issue prescriptions for brand name drug products, but we help patients save a lot of money by dispensing generic equivalents. Another term for "generic equivalent" is "therapeutic equivalent." A brand product contains the same exact active ingredient as the generic. Compared to the brand product, the generic or therapeutic equivalent is equal in terms of strength, quality, performance, safety, intended use, dosage form, route of administration, and rate and extent of absorption... pretty much every category that matters from a medical and scientific perspective. The only difference between a brand product and a generic equivalent is the identity of the manufacturer and the quantity and identity of inactive ingredients (e.g. fillers, binders, and color additives).

How do you determine that a generic drug product is therapeutically equivalent to a brand name drug product?
Pharmacy computer software usually contains this information, but you can also get it from the Federal Orange Book. In the Federal Orange Book, the generic drug product will have a "TE Code" (Therapeutic Equivalence Code) that begins with the letter "A." Pharmacists commonly refer to drug products with this code as "A-rated generics."

What is the official title for the Federal Orange Book?
"Approved Drug Products with Therapeutic Equivalence Evaluations"

A prescription for Lipitor® is given to you verbally over the telephone. Should you dispense the brand name Lipitor or the generic equivalent atorvastatin?
Atorvastatin. You would only dispense the brand name if the prescriber (or his/her agent) expressly said that the brand name is necessary and substitution is not allowed.

What is a narrow therapeutic index drug?
A drug that requires careful dose titration and patient monitoring in order to be used safely and effectively. One of the two following criteria must apply:

- There is less than a 2-fold difference between the median lethal dose (LD50) and the median effective dose (ED50).
- There is less than a 2-fold difference between the minimum toxic concentration (MTC) and the minimum effective concentration (MEC).

Note: ED50 is the dose that produces the desired effect in 50% of the population, and LD50 is the dose that is lethal in 50% of the population.

True or false. A brand name drug with a narrow therapeutic index should not be substituted with a generic drug.
It depends. The pharmacist, using professional judgment combined with knowledge of state laws and regulations, makes the final determination in any generic substitution decision.

PROFESSIONALS WITH PRESCRIBING AUTHORITY

There are two categories of prescribing authority: full authority and limited authority. Four groups of healthcare professionals have full prescribing authority: licensed physicians, dentists, podiatrists, and veterinarians. These practitioners can prescribe any medication as long as they are acting *within their scope of practice*. The "within their scope of practice" part is important. This means that a veterinarian can only prescribe medications to animals, and not to humans; dentists cannot prescribe medication for a medical condition unrelated to the teeth or the oral cavity, etc. See below for a list of professionals with full prescribing authority.

Physicians
Doctor of Medicine (MD)
Doctor of Osteopathic Medicine (DO)

Podiatrists
Doctor of Podiatric Medicine (DPM)

Dentists
Doctor of Dental Medicine (DMD)
Doctor of Dental Surgery (DDS)

Veterinarians
Doctor of Veterinary Medicine (DVM)

Optometrists and midlevel practitioners have limited prescribing authority. Depending on the state they practice in, optometrists have certain restrictions and/or limitations on what they can prescribe, especially when it comes to controlled substances. The same is true for midlevel practitioners, such as physician assistants and nurse practitioners. Additionally, midlevel practitioners can only prescribe specific medications as outlined in a signed, written agreement between them and their supervising physician. A licensed physician must approve every prescription written by a midlevel practitioner.

Optometrists
Doctor of Optometry (OD)

Midlevel Practitioners
Physician Assistant (PA)
Nurse Practitioner (NP)

Note: Some states grant limited prescribing authority to additional groups of qualified health professionals, such as certified nurse midwives, certified registered nurse anesthetists, chiropractors, and even registered pharmacists.

PRESCRIBER IDENTIFICATION NUMBERS

PRESCRIBER IDENTIFIER ABBREVIATIONS

ABBREVIATION	MEANING
DEA number	Drug Enforcement Administration registration number
NPI number	National Provider Identifier number
UPIN	Unique Prescriber Identification Number

OUT WITH THE UPIN, AND IN WITH THE NPI NUMBER

The National Provider Identifier (NPI) number is a unique, 10-digit number used to identify individual prescribers for insurance claim submission/billing purposes. As of 2007, the Health Insurance Portability and Accountability Act (HIPAA) requires all healthcare providers to have an NPI number. HIPAA also requires every insurance company (both government and private) to accept NPI numbers as the standard identifier for financial transactions. Prior to 2007, each prescriber was required to use a number called a Unique Prescriber Identification Number (UPIN) when filing claims with Medicare. Private insurance companies often imposed different identification requirements. Since prescriber identification requirements varied from one insurance company to another, filing claims was more complicated. The rationale behind the NPI number mandate was to standardize and simplify the process of filing insurance claims. Since HIPAA imposed the NPI number requirement in 2007, the UPIN has become obsolete.

WHERE TO FIND NPI NUMBERS

Most prescribers have their NPI number preprinted on the face of their prescriptions. In some states, the law requires this number to appear on each prescription. When the NPI number of a prescriber is unknown by the pharmacy, the pharmacy technician can find the number by performing a search at www.NPInumberlookup.org. In some cases, the technician may need to contact the prescriber's office to ask for the NPI number; for instance, if the prescriber's name is not legible on the prescription, or if the prescriber's last name recently changed and the NPI registration has not been updated to reflect the change.

DEA NUMBERS FOR CONTROLLED SUBSTANCE PRESCRIPTIONS

Another prescriber identification number, the DEA number, is also required when dispensing controlled substances (see pages 32 – 35 for a list of controlled substances). Unlike the NPI number, which HIPAA mandates for all prescribers, not every prescriber is required to have a DEA number. Only practitioners that prescribe controlled substances are required to have a DEA number. To obtain a DEA number, the prescriber must register with the Drug Enforcement Administration. Once registered, prescribers must include their DEA number on the face of every controlled substance prescription they write. Any entity that handles controlled substances is also required to register with the DEA, including drug manufacturers, distributors, research labs, hospitals, and pharmacies.

CHILD-RESISTANT PACKAGING

What law requires child-resistant packaging for drug products?
The Poison Prevention Packaging Act (PPPA) of 1970.

How does the Poison Prevention Packaging Act change the way we dispense drugs?
To comply with this law, pharmacies now dispense prescription in bottles/vials with child-safety caps. There are a few exceptions; including nitroglycerin sublingual tablets and birth control pills.

Why are nitroglycerin sublingual tablets exempt from the PPPA?
Nitroglycerin sublingual tablets are used to restore blood flow to the heart during an exacerbation of angina (characterized by acute, severe chest pain), preventing a potential myocardial infarction (heart attack). Child resistant packaging may cause an individual on the verge of a heart attack to struggle with opening a container of this potentially life-saving medication (nitroglycerin). As a result, this medication is exempt from the rules of the PPPA.

What is the intent of the PPPA?
To protect children from serious injury or illness caused by handling, using, or ingesting medications and other potentially harmful household substances.

How does the PPPA affect drug manufacturers?
The PPPA requires manufacturers to place drug products in packaging that is *significantly difficult* for children under the age of 5 years old to open, yet not difficult for normal adults to open.

What if an adult patient has difficulty with or is unable to open a child safety cap (e.g. due to arthritis)?
Upon request from the patient, a pharmacy can replace the standard child-safety cap with an easy-open cap (also referred to as a “snap cap”).

ROLE OF GOVERNMENT AGENCIES

State Board of Pharmacy
Each state has its own board of pharmacy that is responsible for protecting the health, safety, and welfare of its citizens in matters related to the practice of pharmacy. This is accomplished through the enforcement of pharmacy laws and regulations. State boards of pharmacy are also in charge of regulating traditional compounding pharmacies.

Food and Drug Administration (FDA)
The FDA enforces drug manufacturing laws and regulates prescription drug advertising, which is known as "direct to consumer" (DTC) advertising. The FDA also regulates large-scale compounding facilities.

Drug Enforcement Administration (DEA)
The DEA enforces the federal Controlled Substances Act (CSA) and makes decisions regarding the classification of certain drugs as controlled substances.

Occupational Safety and Health Administration (OSHA)
OSHA enforces occupational health and safety laws. They play a major role in reducing the risk of employee exposure to blood borne pathogens. This is particularly relevant for places where employees routinely work with needles, as is the case in pharmacies with a clean room or pharmacies that offer immunizations and vaccinations.

Federal Trade Commission (FTC)
The FTC regulates advertising for over-the-counter drugs, medical devices, cosmetics, and food products.

Note: The government classifies vitamins and herbal supplements as "food products."

MANUFACTURER DRUG PACKAGE LABELING

This section pertains to stock bottle labeling for prescription drugs. The labeling on a stock container provides information for the pharmacist regarding not only the contents, but also dosage and use information for safe and effective prescribing. From a pharmacy perspective, the most important elements of labeling are 1) the manufacturer's drug package label, which is the label affixed to the stock bottle or container, and 2) the package insert, also commonly referred to as the prescribing information. The exam may test your ability to locate certain information. For instance, where can you find the expiration date? Where can you find information on dosage and administration? Study the outline below to familiarize yourself with the categories of information that appear on the manufacturer's drug package label.

THE CONTENTS ON A MANUFACTURER'S DRUG PACKAGE LABEL

- Brand drug name*
- Generic drug name
- Name and location of the manufacturer, packer, or distributor
- Drug strength or concentration
- Type of dosage form
- Total weight, volume, or number of dosage units contained in the package
- The statement "caution: federal law prohibits dispensing without a prescription" or "Rx Only"
- A statement that refers individuals to the prescribing information (the package insert) for more information
- Storage instructions
- National Drug Code (NDC number) with barcode**
- Expiration date
- Lot number
- A symbol representing the controlled substance schedule in which the drug is listed (i.e. CII, CIII, CIV, or CV)***

*For brand name products only. Does not apply to generics.

**NDC numbers are recommended, but not required.

***For controlled substances only.

Note: The FDA recommends that manufacturers obtain and include an NDC number on the drug package label, but this is not a requirement. Manufacturers are aware that pharmacies rely heavily on NDC numbers when purchasing medications and maintaining inventory records, so it is in the manufacturers' best interest to include an NDC number on the label. Only in very rare cases will you see a drug package label without an NDC number.

EXAMPLE

MANUFACTURER DRUG PACKAGE LABEL

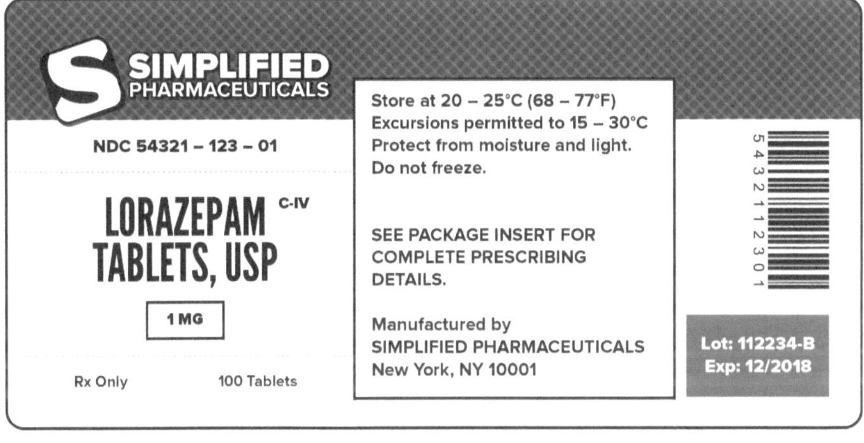

THE CONTENTS ON A PACKAGE INSERT (PRESCRIBING INFORMATION)

Most manufacturers fold the package insert into a small square and glue it to the cap on the stock prescription bottle. The information on the package insert must be unbiased and scientific. The information in the package insert is for healthcare professionals, not patients or consumers. The FDA requires certain information to appear on a package insert. In 2001, the requirements changed. The information included on the package insert will depend on when the drug received FDA-approval. Memorizing all of this information is not necessary. The important thing is that you have a general idea about where to find certain information.

Package Insert Information Requirements for Drugs Approved Before* June 30, 2001:

- Description
- Clinical Pharmacology
- Indications and Usage
- Contraindications
- Warnings
- Precautions
- Adverse Reactions
- Drug Abuse and Dependence**
- Overdosage
- Dosage and Administration
- How Supplied
- Animal Pharmacology/Toxicology
- Clinical Studies
- References

* Drugs approved by the FDA prior to 6/30/2001 are not required to conform to the updated labeling requirements outlined below, but conformance is recommended/encouraged.

**Sections that clearly do not apply need not be included on the package insert. For instance, the section titled "Drug Abuse and Dependence" need not appear on the package insert of a non-controlled substance medication.

Package Insert Information Requirements for Drugs Approved On or After June 30, 2001:

- Boxed Warning
- Indications and Usage
- Dosage and Administration
- Dosage Forms and Strengths
- Contraindications
- Warnings and Precautions
- Adverse Reactions
- Drug Interactions
- Use in Specific Populations
- Drug Abuse and Dependence
- Overdosage
- Description
- Clinical Pharmacology
- Nonclinical Toxicology
- Clinical Studies
- References
- How Supplied/Storage & Handling
- Patient Counseling Information

OVER-THE-COUNTER DRUG PACKAGE LABELING

You also need to be familiar with the different categories of information found on an over-the-counter (OTC) drug package label. As we have mentioned in other sections, OTC medications, unlike prescription medications, are therapeutic agents that customers can purchase without a prescription. Examples include Tums®, Tylenol®, Motrin®, Mucinex®, Prilosec®, and Prevacid®... just to name a few. For our list of the top 45 OTC drugs, see pages 121 – 122.

To get the most out of reviewing this section, we recommend that you retrieve an OTC medication from your drug cabinet at home. If you do not have any OTC medication in your house, then can use the back of your tube of fluoride toothpaste. It will be close enough. Study the label and compare it to the outline below.

OTC DRUG PACKAGE LABEL INFORMATION

- Drug Facts
    - Active Ingredient(s) and strength or concentration per dosage unit.
    - Purpose(s).
- Uses
    - A list of the approved indications/uses.
- Warnings
    - Statements regarding allergies, use in pregnancy and breast-feeding, overdose, drug interactions, age-related warnings, and when to consult a doctor or pharmacist. The statement, "Keep out of reach of children."
- Directions
    - Specific instructions based on age, recommended dose, frequency of dosing and maximum daily dose. For example, the directions for Tylenol® Extra Strength may say, "Adults and children age 12 years and older: take 1 – 2 tablets up to every 6 hours while symptoms last. Do not exceed 6 tablets in a 24-hour period, unless directed by a doctor.
- Other Information
    - Storage requirements.
    - Details regarding electrolyte content (if applicable).
- Inactive Ingredients
    - List of ingredients that do not affect therapeutic action, such as flavoring agents, colorants, and preservatives.
- Contact Information
    - Company name, location, and phone number of the manufacturer.
- Statement regarding the integrity of the tamper-evident packaging, such as "Do not use if safety seal is broken or missing" *
- Expiration date and lot number**

* The FDA requires tamper-evident packaging for most OTC medications. This requirement was established after the 1982 Chicago Tylenol Murders, where someone obtained Tylenol, then laced the capsules with cyanide and returned the bottles to the shelf, leading to the death of seven people.

** If you are following along with a tube of fluoride toothpaste, the expiration date and lot number can be hard to see. It is usually stamped into the crimped end of the tube.

DRUGS & DRUG THERAPY

DOSAGE FORMS

Drug products are available in a variety of dosage forms. The dosage form is essentially the vehicle that delivers the drug to the site of action or the site of absorption. For a drug that acts locally, such as topical creams for conditions of the skin or ophthalmic drops for conditions of the eye, the manufacturer uses a dosage form that delivers the drug directly to the site of action. For drugs that exert their effect at some location inside the body, the manufacturer uses a dosage form that delivers the drug to a site of absorption (usually the gastrointestinal tract) where the drug enters the blood stream. Manufacturers also select dosage forms based on answers to the following types of questions:

Does the drug dissolve in a liquid medium?

o Yes:	Liquid Dosage Form
o No:	Solid Dosage Form or Liquid Suspension

Does the drug dissolve better in water, alcohol, or oil?

o Water:	Suspension or Syrup
o Alcohol:	Elixir or Tincture
o Oil:	Emulsion

Does the drug irritate the lining of the stomach?

o Yes:	Enteric-Coated Tablet or Delayed-Release Tablet or Capsule
o No:	Regular Tablet or Capsule

Do we want the patient to be able to break the doses into fractions?

o Yes:	Scored Tablet
o No:	Regular Tablet

From what location do we want the drug to be absorbed?

o The Stomach and Intestines:	Tablet, Capsule, Suspension, or Solution
o The Intestines Only:	Enteric-Coated Tablet, Delayed-Release Tablet or Capsule
o The Mouth:	Sublingual Tablet or Buccal Lozenge
o The Skin:	Transdermal Patch
o The Rectum:	Rectal Suppository

For locally acting drugs, where will the patient apply the medication?

o The Skin:	Cream, Ointment, Gel, or Lotion
o The Nose:	Nasal Spray
o The Eye:	Ophthalmic Drop
o The Ear:	Otic Drop
o The Lungs:	Inhaler or Nebulizer Solution

LIQUID DOSAGE FORMS

Solution – A solute and a solvent; the solute molecules dissolve to form a homogeneous, single-phase mixture with the solvent.
General Example: salt water
Pharmaceutical Example: the liquid in an EpiPen® (epinephrine solution for injection)

Syrup – Highly concentrated water-based sugar solutions.
General Example: maple syrup
Pharmaceutical Example: ipecac syrup

CONTAINS ALCOHOL

Elixir – Solutions containing water, alcohol, and sweetener.
General Example: certain mixed alcoholic drinks (alcohol, ice/water, and sugar)
Pharmaceutical Example: Lortab® Elixir (hydrocodone/acetaminophen oral solution)

Tincture – Usually alcoholic extracts of crude materials. Alcohol content generally ranges from 15 – 80% for tinctures.
General Example: tincture of iodine
Pharmaceutical Example: Paregoric® (camphorated tincture of opium)

SHAKE WELL

Suspension – A mixture of particles dispersed in a fluid medium; the particles do not dissolve, so the mixture is two-phase.*
General Example: sand in water
Pharmaceutical Example: Mycostatin® (nystatin oral suspension)

Emulsion – A mixture in which one liquids is suspended in another.
General Example: oil in water
Pharmaceutical Example: Restasis® (cyclosporine ophthalmic emulsion)

*Two-phase mixtures (i.e. suspensions and emulsions) must be shaken prior to dispensing and before each dose to ensure the medication is evenly distributed throughout the liquid medium. To alert the patient to this fact, you should place a "shake well" auxiliary label on the bottle of any suspension or emulsion you dispense. To understand the importance of this concept, look at the illustration below. Imagine that the drug is represented by the gray phase. If the patient does not "shake well," then the patient will receive less drug in the first few doses and much more drug in the last few doses.

ILLUSTRATION: WHY SUSPENSIONS & EMULSIONS MUST BE SHAKEN

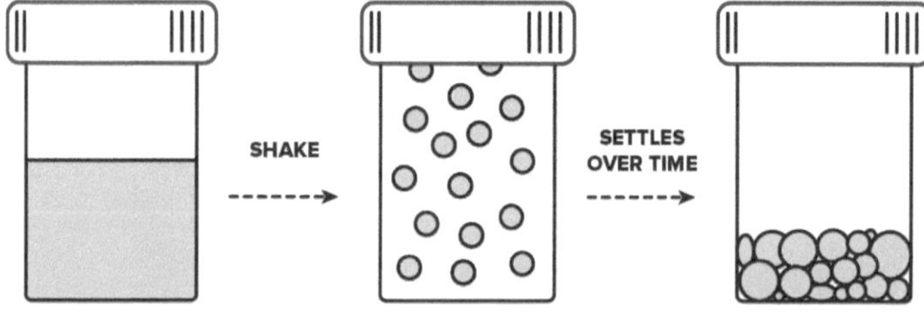

SOLID DOSAGE FORMS

Tablet

A powdery mixture of an active pharmaceutical ingredient and excipients (inert/inactive ingredients, such as fillers, binders, and colorants) pressed into a disc or other small shape. Tablets are the most popular dosage form.

Scored Tablet

Certain tablets should never be broken. For instance, most extended-release tablets and capsules *must* be swallowed whole because splitting them can destroy the slow release mechanism and cause an overdose. On the other hand, some tablets are designed by the manufacturer with an indentation (i.e. they are "scored") to make it easy for the patient to divide the tablet into fractions. Below is an illustration of two scored tablets. On the left, we see a tablet that is scored into equal quarters. On the right, we see a tablet that is scored into equal halves. The illustration shows the top view of the tablet and the side view (rotated 90 degrees on the dashed-line axis) to better illustrate the indentation.

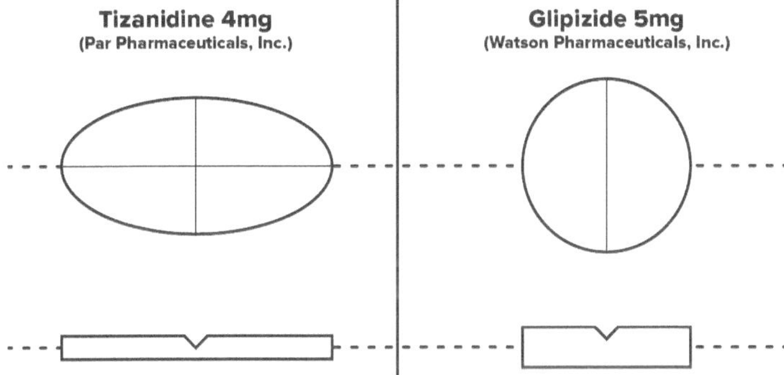

Enteric-Coated (EC) Tablet

An enteric coating is composed of special material that will not dissolve in the acidic environment of the stomach, but will dissolve in the more neutral environment of the small intestines. As a result, when enteric-coated tablets are ingested, they do not dissolve until after they pass through the stomach and enter the small intestine. Manufacturers apply this coating for medications that would otherwise irritate or damage the lining of the stomach. An example is enteric-coated aspirin.

SWALLOW WHOLE DO NOT CRUSH OR CHEW

Sublingual (SL) Tablet

Sublingual tablets dissolve under the tongue, delivering medication across the tissue beneath the tongue, directly into the bloodstream. By entering the bloodstream directly, the drug can exert is pharmacologic effect much faster. A great example is the nitroglycerin sublingual tablet.

DISSOLVE UNDER TONGUE, DO NOT SWALLOW WHOLE

Orally Disintegrating Tablet (ODT)

Orally disintegrating tablets dissolve in the saliva. They are especially useful for patients that experience difficulty or pain when swallowing. For example, let's say a patient has experienced severe nausea and vomiting. While vomiting, acid from the stomach has damaged the lining of the patient's esophagus, making it painful to swallow. The anti-nausea medication ondansetron is available as an ODT for situations such as this.

DISSOLVE IN MOUTH. DO NOT SWALLOW WHOLE

Capsule

Capsules are composed of two parts: the shell (usually made of hard gelatin) and the contents (drug powder, pellets, or tiny tablets). Many drugs are available in capsule form. Capsules are one of the most popular dosage forms, second only to tablets.

Soft Gelatin Capsule

Also commonly referred to as "gelcaps" or "softgels," this rendition of the capsule is usually yellow or amber and has a relatively transparent shell with liquid contents. Lovaza® and Tessalon® Perles are good examples.

Caplet

Capsule-shaped tablets. Tylenol® Extra Strength and Valtrex® are good examples.

Lozenge

Medicated candies designed to dissolve slowly – and thus release medication slowly – within the oral cavity. A good example is the Cepacol® Sore Throat Lozenge, which delivers benzocaine and menthol directly to the throat area. Clotrimazole is another example, which is available as a "tablet lozenge" for the treatment of oral thrush. Tablet lozenges have the appearance of a tablet, usually white and chalky, but they dissolve in the mouth like a traditional candy lozenge.

Troche

Technically, these are compressed lozenges, but many healthcare professionals use the terms "lozenge" and "troche" interchangeably.

MODIFIED-RELEASE VS IMMEDIATE-RELEASE

Certain medications are available in a standard immediate-release version and a special modified-release version. The immediate-release versions dissolve quickly. Since immediate-release is the default/standard version of a medication, the FDA does not require the drug package label to specify "immediate-release." Otherwise, a vast majority of medications would have this term printed on their label. Another term for immediate-release is "regular-release."

On the other hand, modified-release formulations (i.e. extended-release and delayed-release) have a mechanism that controls the release of medication from the dosage form. Modified release is a broad term that encompasses two possible medication release mechanisms. #1 The "delayed release" mechanism (abbreviated "DR"), which is equivalent to an enteric coating. This mechanism delays the release of the medication until the dosage form (i.e. tablet, capsule, or particulate matter in a liquid suspension) passes through the stomach and enters the small intestine. #2 The "extended-release" mechanism (abbreviated "ER"), which works by slowing the rate of medication release from a dosage form. Several processes have been designed to achieve the extended-release effect, and, for that reason, there are several names and abbreviations that all essentially mean, "extended-release." See the chart below for some common examples.

Modified Release Mechanism	Abbreviation(s)	Example(s)
Controlled Delivery	CD	Metadate CD®
Controlled-Release	CR	Paxil CR®, Ambien CR®
Extended-Release	ER, XL, XR	Depakote® ER, Toprol-XL®, Quillivant XR®
Long-Acting	LA	Detrol® LA
Sustained-Release	SR	Wellbutrin SR®

Note: According to the United States Pharmacopoeia (USP), delayed-release is synonymous with enteric-coated. All other modified-release dosage forms (CD, CR, LA, ER, XL, XR, and SR) employ some version of an extended release (ER) mechanism.

SWALLOW WHOLE
DO NOT CRUSH OR CHEW

SEMI-SOLID DOSAGE FORMS

Semi-solid dosage forms include ointments, creams, gels, and pastes. These dosage forms are most commonly used for topical application (on the skin), but they can also be formulated for application to other sites. Examples include erythromycin ophthalmic ointment, Premarin® vaginal cream, Ayr® saline nasal gel, Proctozone-HC rectal ointment, and Prevident® 5000 Plus toothpaste.

Ointments

Ointments are mixtures of medication in a base of petroleum jelly or something similar to petroleum jelly. Ointments often have a greasy texture and tend to sit on top of the skin. This creates a moisture barrier that can be beneficial for dry skin. Because ointments sit on top of the skin, they deliver medication slower and over a longer period of time compared to other topical dosage forms. An example is Neosporin®.

Creams

Creams are typically medicated emulsions of oil-in-water that are easy to wash off. Compared to ointments, creams are lighter, less sticky, and less greasy. Creams tend to rub into the skin, rather than sit on top as ointments do. Because they rub into the skin, creams release medication faster than ointments. An example is Lotrimin® AF cream.

Gels

Gels are mixtures of medication in a water-based medium. A gelling agent gives the water base a jelly-like consistency. Examples include Finacea® topical gel and Diastat® rectal gel.

Pastes

Pastes are thicker and stiffer than the other semi-solid dosage forms. Because of their thickness, they tend to penetrate the skin poorly, but they are effective skin protectants. The most common place we see paste dosage forms is dental preparations. An example is Biotene® dry mouth toothpaste.

LOTIONS

Lotions

Lotions are typically oil-in-water emulsions in a water-based medium. If you recall, creams are also oil-in-water emulsions. The same characteristic that apply to creams also apply to lotions. For example, they both tend to be less greasy and less sticky compared to ointments. The big difference between a cream and a lotion is the integration of a water-based medium, making lotions thinner and easier to spread. Because lotions are not as thick and stiff as ointments, creams, gels, and pastes, we do not consider them "semi-solids."

INHALATION SOLUTIONS, AEROSOLS, AND POWDERS

There are three major types of inhalable dosage forms: nebulizer solutions, metered dose inhalers, and dry powder inhalers. All of these dosage forms involve administration of drug product by oral inhalation.

Nebulizer Solutions
Medicated solutions that are vaporized via air pressure generated by a machine called a nebulizer. Examples include AccuNeb®, DouNeb®, and Atrovent®.

Metered Dose Inhalers (MDIs)
Handheld devices that propel aerosolized drug particles when actuated. Chlorofluorocarbons (CFCs) were once the propellant of choice for MDIs, but the government outlawed the use of CFCs since they degrade ozone. The new propellant of choice used by manufacturers is the hydrofluoroalkanes (HFAs). Examples include Ventolin® HFA, ProAir® HFA, and Proventil® HFA.

Dry Powder Inhalers
A rather unique type of inhaler. They do not employ propellants. Rather, the medication comes as a powder-filled capsule – the contents of which are inhaled directly into the patient's lungs using capsule-puncturing device equipped with a mouthpiece for inhalation. Examples include Advair® Diskus, Serevent® Diskus, and Spiriva® HandiHaler.

TRANSDERMAL DRUG DELIVERY SYSTEMS

Certain medications have special properties that enable them to cross the skin and enter the bloodstream. When these drugs are manufactured as skin patches, we call them transdermal drug delivery systems. Examples include Transderm Scop® for motion sickness, Ortho Evra® for birth control, Vivelle-Dot® for symptoms of menopause, Nitro-Dur® for angina, and Duragesic® for chronic pain. These dosage forms are known for their convenience. Most patches contain enough medication to last for several days.

SUPPOSITORIES AND INSERTS

Suppositories are solid under refrigeration and, in most cases, at room temperature, but melt at normal body temperature. There are different types of suppositories, but rectal suppositories are the most common. Rectal suppositories deliver medication directly to the rectum for one of two purposes. #1 To remain in the colon for treatment of a local condition, such as hemorrhoid pain or constipation, or #2 To be absorbed from the colon into the blood stream for treatment of a systemic condition, such as a seizure or nausea and vomiting. An example of a rectal suppository for a local condition is the Tucks® suppository for hemorrhoids. For a systemic condition, an example is Phenadoz® suppositories for nausea and vomiting.

A REVIEW OF MAJOR DRUG CLASSES & BASIC PHARMACOLOGY

Drugs are grouped into categories – referred to as "drug classes" – based on their pharmacology. Drugs within the same drug class share the same pharmacologic mechanism of action. Studying the pharmacology of one drug at a time is tedious and inefficient. To simplify and expedite the process, we will study pharmacology one drug class at a time. Assume that the drugs discussed in this section are prescription only unless specified otherwise. Topics covered will include uses (indications), mechanisms of action (pharmacology), side effects, common drug interactions, and other noteworthy details. Focus on brand and generic drug names, indications, and key points.

Understanding High Blood Pressure

High blood pressure (hypertension) is a chronic medical condition. Over the course of many years, the force of high pressure inside the blood vessels causes damage, which creates rough patches. Cholesterol tends to stick to and build up on these rough patches, forming little mounds. We call this process atherosclerosis, and it impedes the flow of blood through the blood vessel, which can cause problems such as coronary artery disease, angina, and myocardial infarction. Hypertension is extremely common, and several drugs are available to treat it.

Understanding ACE Inhibitors and ARBs

WHAT ARE ACE INHIBITORS AND ARBs?

ACE inhibitor is an abbreviation for Angiotensin Converting Enzyme inhibitor. ARB is an abbreviation for Angiotensin Receptor Blocker. These drug classes are very similar. They both reduce the effect of a hormone called angiotensin. What does angiotensin do? It is a vasoconstrictor. Furthermore, an enzyme abbreviated as "ACE" converts angiotensin to an even more powerful blood vessel constricting hormone called angiotensin II, but the story doesn't end there. Angiotensin II goes on to stimulate the release of another hormone called aldosterone, which causes salt retention. Salt retention raises blood pressure further yet. By interfering with angiotensin before it becomes angiotensin II, we prevent a lot of the blood vessel constriction and salt retention that can contribute to high blood pressure. I know, it gets a little complicated, but do not be overwhelmed by all of these details. The take home message is that ACE inhibitors and ARBs share a similar mechanism of action and both drug classes reduce blood pressure.

ACE INHIBITORS VS ARBS... SIDE EFFECT COMPARISON

Because ACE inhibitors and ARBs share a similar mechanism of action, they also have similar side effects. Nonetheless, there are minor differences. Observe the chart below for a comparison of the most common and severe potential side effects.

Side Effect	ACE Inhibitors	ARBs
Nonproductive Cough	✓	
Hypotension	✓	✓
Hyperkalemia	✓	✓
Anaphylaxis	✓	✓

ACE INHIBITORS AND ARBS ARE BOTH PREGNANCY CATEGORY X NEVER TO BE USED DURING PREGNANCY

ANGIOTENSIN CONVERTING ENZYME (ACE) INHIBITORS FOR HYPERTENSION

BRAND NAME	GENERIC NAME
Lotensin®	Benazepril
Vasotec®	Enalapril
Prinivil®, Zestril®	Lisinopril
Accupril®	Quinapril
Altace®	Ramipril

**Note: notice how the generic names of the ACE inhibitors end in "–pril."*

BACKGROUND: Angiotensin is a hormone produced by the kidneys. It causes vasoconstriction and salt retention, which contribute to high blood pressure.

PHARMACOLOGY: ACE inhibitors reduce the effect of angiotensin, ultimately lowering blood pressure by relaxing the blood vessels and preventing salt retention.

INDICATIONS: Hypertension, Heart Failure, Myocardial Infarction (Heart Attack), Kidney Protection in Diabetic Patients

SIDE EFFECTS: Nonproductive Cough, Hypotension, Hyperkalemia, Anaphylaxis (rare)

DRUG INTERACTIONS: ACE inhibitors can cause high potassium, which can lead to life-threatening cardiac arrhythmias. Patients using potassium supplements or potassium-sparing diuretics are more likely to experience problems.

NOTES: ACE inhibitors cause birth defects and should never be used during pregnancy (pregnancy category X). About 20% of patients on ACE inhibitors experience a dry, nonproductive cough. The only way to eliminate this side effect is to discontinue the ACE inhibitor. Switch to an ARB for the same pharmacologic effect without the dry cough side effect.

DO NOT USE IF YOU ARE PREGNANT

A COMMON SIDE EFFECT AMONG BLOOD PRESSURE DRUGS

One thing you should notice about drugs that lower blood pressure is that they can all potentially cause hypotension (low blood pressure). This happens when we get too much of the desired effect.

Symptoms of hypotension include fatigue, dizziness, blurred vision, and, in severe cases, loss of consciousness – all of which are consequences of insufficient blood flow to the brain.

ANGIOTENSIN RECEPTOR BLOCKERS (ARBs) FOR HYPERTENSION

BRAND NAME	GENERIC NAME
Edarbi®	Azilsartan
Atacand®	Candesartan
Avapro®	Irbesartan
Cozaar®	Losartan
Benicar®	Olmesartan
Micardis®	Telmisartan
Diovan®	Valsartan

**Note: notice how the generic names of the ARBs all end in "–sartan."*

BACKGROUND: For angiotensin to exert its effect, it must be able to bind to angiotensin receptors.

PHARMACOLOGY: ARBs reduce the effect of angiotensin by preventing receptor binding; ultimately lowering blood pressure by relaxing the blood vessels and reducing salt retention.

INDICATIONS: Hypertension, Heart Failure, Myocardial Infarction (Heart Attack) Stroke Prevention, Renal Protection in Diabetic Patients

SIDE EFFECTS: Fatigue, Dizziness, Hyperkalemia, Hypotension, Anaphylaxis (rare).

DRUG INTERACTIONS: Since ARBs can increase potassium levels, potassium supplements and potassium-sparing diuretics can increase the risk of hyperkalemia.

NOTES: As with the ACE inhibitors, ARBs cause birth defects and should never be used during pregnancy (pregnancy category X).

DO NOT USE IF YOU ARE PREGNANT

WHAT EXACTLY IS URINE?

The kidneys work as filters for circulating blood. As the heart pumps blood back and forth through arteries and veins, the kidneys continuously function to remove waste products from the blood, producing urine. Everything that ends up in the urine was once a part of the blood. This includes water, electrolytes, metabolized vitamins, and even medications.

KIDNEYS AND ELECTROLYTES

Nutrients and water from food and beverages pass from the intestinal tract into the bloodstream through a process called "absorption." Nutrients include fat, protein, carbohydrates, vitamins and electrolytes (e.g. sodium, potassium, calcium, magnesium). Electrolytes are needed mainly for nerve and muscle function. If electrolyte levels are too low or too high, the consequences can be serious, including seizures, cardiac arrhythmias, and even death. The kidneys constantly work to maintain the proper balance of electrolytes. They accomplish this by diverting electrolytes from the blood into the urine when levels are high and preventing electrolytes from entering the urine when levels in the blood are low.

THE RELATIONSHIP BETWEEN SODIUM AND BLOOD PRESSURE

By a process called osmosis, sodium attracts water. Excess salt (sodium chloride) in the bloodstream causes water retention, and water retention leads to increased blood pressure.

DIURETICS AND SODIUM

Diuretics increase urine production by forcing the kidneys to divert more sodium from the blood into the urine. By osmosis, water follows sodium into the urine. When water leaves the blood, the blood takes up less space in the blood vessels, and this causes blood pressure to drop.

DIURETICS AND POTASSIUM

There are three classes of diuretics: 1) Thiazide Diuretics, 2) Loop Diuretics and 3) Potassium-Sparing Diuretics. Diuretics remove sodium from the blood, but they also remove potassium. This is a side effect, and it frequently leads to low potassium levels. Potassium-sparing diuretics are the exception. They remove sodium without removing potassium.

THIAZIDE DIURETICS FOR HYPERTENSION

BRAND NAME	GENERIC NAME
Hygroton®, Thalitone®	Chlorthalidone
Microzide®	Hydrochlorothiazide

BACKGROUND: Sodium, found in salt, is associated with water retention and, consequently, hypertension.

PHARMACOLOGY: Thiazide diuretics increase the transfer of salt and water from blood to urine, thus reducing blood pressure.

INDICATIONS: Hypertension, Edema

SIDE EFFECTS: Hypotension, Hypokalemia, Hyperuricemia, Muscle Cramps (caused by low potassium), Cardiac Arrhythmias (also caused by low potassium), Photosensitivity (predisposition to sunburn), SJS (rare)

DRUG INTERACTIONS: Potential for severe hypotension when combined with other blood pressure-lowering drugs (ACE inhibitors, ARBs, loop diuretics, etc.). Also, potential for severe hypokalemia when used with loop diuretics.

NOTES: Thiazides share a similarity with sulfonamide antibiotics... not in their mechanism of action, but in their chemical structure. Because of this similarity, patients with a sulfa allergy may also be allergic to thiazide diuretics.

POTASSIUM REPLACEMENT WITH THIAZIDE AND LOOP DIURETICS

As we have discussed, thiazide diuretics and loop diuretics deplete potassium. For this reason, many prescribers will take measures to prevent hypokalemia in patients taking one or both of these diuretics. Expect to see one or more of the following strategies:

1. The prescriber instruct patient to "take with a banana or orange juice"
2. The prescriber issues a potassium supplement (K-Dur®, Klor-Con®)
3. The prescriber issues a combination drug product (discussed below)

Note: Bananas and orange juice are naturally high in potassium.

HYDROCHLOROTHIAZIDE COMBINATION PRODUCTS

Manufacturers produce several thiazide-ARB and thiazide-ACE inhibitor combinations for a couple of reasons: #1 Most patients require more than one hypertension drug to achieve their blood pressure goal, and #2 ARBs and ACE inhibitors can oppose the potassium-depleting effect of thiazide diuretics. See the two most popular combinations below.

BRAND NAME	GENERIC NAME
Zestoretic®	Lisinopril/Hydrochlorothiazide
Hyzaar®	Losartan/Hydrochlorothiazide

LOOP DIURETICS FOR HYPERTENSION

BRAND NAME	GENERIC NAME
Bumex®	Bumetanide
Edecrin®	Ethacrynic Acid
Lasix®	Furosemide
Demadex®	Torsemide

BACKGROUND: Sodium, found in salt, is associated with water retention & hypertension.

PHARMACOLOGY: Similar to thiazide diuretics, loop diuretics promote the transfer of salt and water from the blood to the urine, thus reducing blood pressure.

INDICATIONS: Hypertension, Edema

SIDE EFFECTS: Hypokalemia, Hypotension, Muscle Cramps (caused by low potassium), Cardiac Arrhythmias (caused by low potassium), Photosensitivity (predisposition to sunburn), SJS (rare)

DRUG INTERACTIONS: Virtually the same drug interactions as seen with the thiazide diuretics – additive hypotension when combined with other drugs that can cause hypotension, and additive hypokalemia when administered with thiazide diuretics.

NOTES: Loop diuretics are the most effective diuretics available. Loop diuretics have the potential to cause life-threatening potassium depletion if used improperly.

MNEMONIC FOR LOOP DIURETIC GENERIC NAMES

"BEAU-TI-FUL"

When you breakdown the word "beautiful" into its three syllables (beau-ti-ful), you see that each syllable begins with a letter corresponding to the first letter of the generic name of the most commonly used loop diuretics (bumetanide, torsemide, and furosemide).

The "**B**" in **B**eau- corresponds to the "**B**" in **B**umetanide.
The "**T**" in -**T**i- corresponds to the "**T**" in **T**orsemide.
The "**F**" in –**F**ul corresponds to the "**F**" in **F**urosemide.

EXPECT UNIQUE INSTRUCTIONS FROM TIME TO TIME

Since prescribers may issue loop diuretics to treat edema in patients with heart failure, you will occasionally see odd-looking instructions. For instance, "take 1 tablet by mouth once daily if weight increases > 2 pounds in 24 hours." Why? Rapid weight gain is usually a sign of fluid retention ("water weight"), which causes serious problems in heart failure.

POTASSIUM-SPARING DIURETICS
FOR HYPERTENSION

BRAND NAME	GENERIC NAME
Midamor®	Amiloride
Inspra®	Eplerenone
Aldactone®	Spironolactone
Dyrenium®	Triamterene

BACKGROUND: Hypokalemia is a common side effect caused by diuretics.

PHARMACOLOGY: Increase the amount of salt and water that leaves the body via the urine, but without causing low potassium.

INDICATIONS: Hypertension, Heart Failure

SIDE EFFECTS: Hyperkalemia, Hypotension

DRUG INTERACTIONS: Because these drugs work specifically to prevent potassium loss, they can actually cause high potassium levels in the blood (hyperkalemia). The use of potassium supplements increases the risk of hyperkalemia.

NOTES: Potassium-sparing diuretics have a mechanism that does not work quite as well as the thiazide or loop diuretics, but, as their name suggests, they have a mechanism that does not lead to the loss of potassium. In fact, potassium-sparing diuretics can actually cause potassium levels to increase. For this reason, when patients need more than one medication to achieve their blood pressure goal, one option prescribers may use is to combine a potassium-sparing diuretic with a thiazide diuretic. This induces diuresis and lowers blood pressure by two different mechanisms, and, since they have opposing effects on potassium levels, it helps prevent potassium imbalances as well. Note the combination drugs below.

POTASSIUM-SPARING–THIAZIDE DIURETIC COMBINATION DRUGS

BRAND NAME	GENERIC NAME
Aldactazide®	Spironolactone/Hydrochlorothiazide
Dyazide®, Maxzide®	Triamterene/Hydrochlorothiazide

Understanding Alpha and Beta Receptors

BLOOD VESSELS HAVE MUSCLE

The cardiovascular system is composed of the heart and blood vessels. The blood vessels provide a structural, tube-like network to channel blood to and from every living part of the body, and the heart provides the force needed to circulate the blood through the vessels. You may already know that the heart is a muscle, but did you know that blood vessels are lined with muscle as well? The muscle in blood vessels will constrict to limit blood flow and relax to increase blood flow. For example, when you are engaged in vigorous physical activity, the blood vessels carrying blood to the intestines will contract, while the blood vessels that carry blood to the skeletal muscles will expand. Why do we care? We care, because blood vessel constriction increases blood pressure and blood vessel relaxation decreases blood pressure. Furthermore, we can control these processes pharmacologically.

ALPHA$_1$, ALPHA$_2$, AND BETA RECEPTORS... WHAT ARE THEY?

All of these receptors are associated with the cardiovascular system (the heart and blood vessels). Alpha$_1$ & alpha$_2$ receptors help regulate blood pressure by constricting and relaxing the blood vessels located all throughout the body. Beta-receptors are involved in regulating how fast and hard the heartbeats, which also has an effect on blood pressure. Beta-receptor activation also expands/opens the airways.

ALPHA$_1$ RECEPTORS

Activation of alpha$_1$ receptors causes blood vessel constriction, which raises blood pressure. The body uses adrenaline & norepinephrine to activate these receptors.

ALPHA$_2$ RECEPTORS

Activation of alpha$_2$ receptors leads to reduced adrenaline & norepinephrine levels, consequently reducing blood pressure.

BETA RECEPTORS

Activation of beta-receptors causes the heart to beat faster and harder, which raises blood pressure. Activation of beta-receptors also causes the airways in the lungs to open up. Blocking beta-receptor activity will cause the heart to relax and has a blood pressure-lowering effect. Some beta-receptor blockers can cause breathing problems for patients with asthma/COPD.

ALPHA$_1$ RECEPTOR ANTAGONISTS (ALPHA$_1$ BLOCKERS) FOR HYPERTENSION

BRAND NAME	GENERIC NAME
Uroxatral®	Afluzosin
Cardura®	Doxazosin
Rapaflo®	Silodosin
Flomax®	Tamsulosin
Hytrin®	Terazosin

**Note: notice how the generic names of the aplha$_1$-blockers all end in "–osin."*

BACKGROUND: Activation of alpha$_1$ receptors causes blood vessels to constrict.

PHARMACOLOGY: Prevent activation of alpha$_1$ receptors, leading to relaxation of blood vessels. These drugs also happen to relax muscles in the bladder neck and prostate, which is why drugs from this class can also be used to treat enlarged prostate (BPH).

INDICATIONS: Hypertension, Benign Prostatic Hyperplasia (BPH)

SIDE EFFECTS: Orthostatic Hypotension (blood pressure drops quickly upon changing from the sitting position to standing), Dizziness, Syncope

DRUG INTERACTIONS: Increased risk of hypotension when used with other blood pressure lowering drugs.

NOTES: Benign prostatic hyperplasia is a condition in where we see enlargement of the prostate gland. The main symptom is obstruction of urinary outflow. There are alpha$_1$ receptors in the prostate and in the neck of the bladder, which is located next to the prostate. By blocking alpha$_1$ receptors, the muscle in the prostate and bladder neck relax, allowing urine to flow out unobstructed. Alpha$_1$ blockers also relax blood vessels all throughout the body. Some of these drugs target BPH, others high blood pressure.

EMERGENCY ANAPHYLAXIS

People with a severe allergy, such as to bee stings, often carry an EpiPen®. An EpiPen® is an auto-injector device containing epinephrine (adrenaline), which patients inject into their thigh during an anaphylactic reaction. During anaphylaxis, patients typically have dangerously low blood pressure and severe difficulty breathing. The active ingredient in the EpiPen®, epinephrine, stimulates both alpha and beta-receptors, leading to blood vessel constriction, stronger and faster heart beats, and dilation of the airways. While EpiPen is the most popular device of its kind, other brands exist. See below.

BRAND NAME	GENERIC NAME
Auvi-Q®	Epinephrine
Twinject®	Epinephrine

ALPHA$_2$ RECEPTOR AGONISTS (ALPHA$_2$ AGONISTS) FOR HYPERTENSION

BRAND NAME	GENERIC NAME
Catapress®, Kapvay®	Clonidine
Intuniv®, Tenex®	Guanfacine
Aldomet®	Methyldopa

BACKGROUND: The nervous system releases norepinephrine all the time. More in times of stress, less in times of rest, but there is always some level of norepinephrine present. To prevent too much norepinephrine from releasing at one time, our nerve cells have regulators known as alpha$_2$ receptors. Consider this analogy... A thermostat is to heat from a furnace as alpha$_2$ receptors are to norepinephrine from the nervous system. When the temperature in a room gets too high, the thermostat signals the furnace to stop releasing heat. Likewise, when the norepinephrine levels in a body get too high, alpha$_2$ receptors signal the nervous system to stop releasing norepinephrine.

PHARMACOLOGY: Activate aplha$_2$ receptors, causing a decrease in norepinephrine levels. This ultimately has a blood pressure- lowering effect.

INDICATIONS: Hypertension, ADHD

SIDE EFFECTS: Bradycardia, Rebound Hypertension (high blood pressure that occurs when the medication is withdrawn)

DRUG INTERACTIONS: Increased risk of hypotension when used with other drugs that decrease blood pressure. Increased risk of bradycardia when used with drugs that decrease heart rate (e.g. beta-blockers).

NOTES: Rebound hypertension is high blood pressure that occurs when patients abruptly stop taking certain blood pressure medications – a symptom of medication withdrawal. The pharmacist can advise patients wishing to discontinue a medication. If a patient asks about how to discontinue a medication, refer them to the pharmacist or their physician.

BETA RECEPTOR ANTAGONISTS (BETA-BLOCKERS) FOR HYPERTENSION

BRAND NAME	GENERIC NAME
Sectral®	Acebutalol
Tenormin®	Atenolol
Coreg®	Carvedilol
Trandate®	Labetalol
Toprol XL®	Metoprolol succinate (extended-release)
Lopressor®	Metoprolol tartrate (immediate-release)
Inderal®	Propranolol
Betapace®	Sotalol

**Note: notice how the generic names of most of the beta-blockers end in "–olol."*

BACKGROUND: Beta-receptor activation increases heart rate, increases the force of heartbeats, and dilates the airways in the lungs.

PHARMACOLOGY: Prevent activation of beta-receptors, reducing the heart rate and reducing the force of heartbeats. Beta-blockers also relax the blood vessels. These effects lead to decreased blood pressure and heart rate.

INDICATIONS: Hypertension, Angina, Atrial Fibrillation, Myocardial Infarction, Migraine Prevention

SIDE EFFECTS: Bradycardia, Exacerbation of Asthma or COPD, Hypotension, Fatigue

DRUG INTERACTIONS: Certain beta-blockers can interfere with the effect of some asthma medications, like albuterol, that work by activating beta-receptors. The risk of hypotension increases when combined with other drugs that lower blood pressure.

NOTES: Abrupt cessation of a beta-blocker can cause serious withdrawal symptoms. If a patient suddenly stops taking a beta-blocker, they can have a heart attack. If a patient mentions anything about stopping a medication on his/her own, alert the pharmacist.

THE MANY USES OF BETA BLOCKERS

As you can see from the long and diverse list of indications, beta-blockers are versatile. They can treat a variety of conditions, mostly heart-related. I just want to take a second to explain why... Since beta-blockers decrease the rate and force of the heartbeat, they take some stress off the heart... The heart does not have to work as hard. As a result, the heart requires less oxygen. Remember the whole issue with angina and heart attacks is that the heart is not receiving enough oxygen. Beta-blockers also relax blood vessels, which is perfect for improving blood flow to an oxygen-deprived heart. Atrial fibrillation is another condition where a beta-blocker can be beneficial. Atrial fibrillation is a type of cardiac arrhythmia – the rhythm of the heartbeat is abnormal. One way to normalize the rhythm is to slow down the heart using a beta-blocker.

CALCIUM CHANNEL BLOCKERS (CCBs) FOR HYPERTENSION

BRAND NAME	GENERIC NAME
Norvasc®	Amlodipine
Cardizem®, Tiazac®, Taztia XT®	Diltiazem
Plendil®	Felodipine
Cardene®	Nicardipine
Procardia®	Nifedipine
Sular®	Nisoldipine
Isoptin®, Verelan®, Calan®	Verapamil

BACKGROUND: The muscle tissue that forms the heart and lines blood vessels requires calcium for effective contraction.

PHARMACOLOGY: Reduce the amount of calcium available to cardiac and vascular muscle cells. With less calcium, the heart beats with less force and the blood vessels relax, both leading to a drop in blood pressure.

INDICATIONS: Hypertension, Angina

SIDE EFFECTS: Fatigue, Edema

DRUG INTERACTIONS: The risk of hypotension increases when taken with other drugs that lower blood pressure.

Note: Angina is chest pain resulting from inadequate blood flow to the heart.

Understanding High Cholesterol

Similar to hypertension, high cholesterol is a chronic condition. Cholesterol levels must be high for several years before a negative effect is recognized. The long-term negative effects include coronary artery disease, angina, and myocardial infarction.

THE TWO SOURCES OF CHOLESTEROL

When we think of cholesterol, we often think of fatty food, but cholesterol actually comes from another place as well... the liver! Our livers produce cholesterol to ensure that cholesterol is present even if we are not obtaining it from food. While cholesterol can have negative effects when levels are high, the body needs some cholesterol for important processes like hormone production and cell wall synthesis. The amount of cholesterol produced by the liver varies from person to person depending on genetics.

HMG-CoA REDUCTASE INHIBITORS (STATINS) FOR HIGH CHOLESTEROL

BRAND NAME	GENERIC NAME
Lipitor®	Atorvastatin
Lescol®	Fluvastatin
Mevacor®	Lovastatin
Livalo®	Pitavastatin
Pravachol®	Pravastatin
Crestor®	Rosuvastatin
Zocor®	Simvastatin

**Note: notice how the generic names end in "–statin."*

BACKGROUND: Cholesterol comes from two sources: dietary intake (food) and production by the liver.

PHARMACOLOGY: Inhibit the enzyme HMG-CoA reductase, which is the key enzyme used by the liver to produce cholesterol.

DO NOT USE IF YOU ARE PREGNANT

INDICATIONS: High Cholesterol

SIDE EFFECTS: Muscle Aches, Myopathy

DRUG INTERACTIONS: Grapefruit juice, in large amounts, can interfere with the metabolism and elimination of statins. This can cause statins to accumulate in the body, eventually leading to serious health problems.

NOTES: Statins cause birth defects and should never be used during pregnancy (pregnancy category X). The liver ramps up cholesterol production at night, so statins are generally more effective when administered at night. Certain statins (e.g. atorvastatin and rosuvastatin) are eliminated from the body at a very slow rate. For this reason, it is not necessary to take atorvastatin or rosuvastatin at night; they can be taken at any time of the day. Since HMG-CoA reductase inhibitors only reduce cholesterol production and do not have an effect on dietary intake, patients should make dietary changes to reduce the amount of cholesterol they consume. How? Read nutrition labels. Avoid foods high in saturated fat and cholesterol (doughnuts, Big Macs, fried chicken, etc.).

ALL STATINS ARE PREGNANCY CATEGORY X
NEVER TO BE USED DURING PREGNANCY

BILE ACID SEQUESTRANTS
FOR HIGH CHOLESTEROL

BRAND NAME	GENERIC NAME
Colestid®	Colestipol
Questran®	Cholestyramine
Welchol®	Colesevelam

BACKGROUND: The cholesterol produced by the liver becomes bile acid, which is a thick, fluid mixture that enters the intestinal tract to aid in the absorption of fat.

PHARMACOLOGY: Bind to ("sequester") cholesterol from bile acid, carrying the cholesterol through the intestines and exiting the body during defecation. This prevents cholesterol produced by the liver from entering the bloodstream.

INDICATIONS: High Cholesterol

SIDE EFFECTS: Constipation, Flatulence

DRUG INTERACTIONS: Bile acid sequestrants work by binding to and preventing the absorption of cholesterol from the intestinal tract. Unsurprisingly, this class of drugs can also interfere with the absorption of many other drugs. There are too many drug interactions to list. Generally, patients should separate doses of other drugs by a few hours to prevent drug interactions.

PRESCRIBED OFF-LABEL FOR DIARRHEA

Since this class of medication commonly causes constipation as a side effect, some doctors will prescribe bile acid sequestrants off-label for the treatment of diarrhea.

THE CHOLESTEROL-LOWERING MECHANISM OF ZETIA® IS SIMILAR...

Zetia® (ezetimibe) is a popular cholesterol-lowering drug that works in a way similar to the bile acid sequestrants; however, Zetia® belongs to a drug class of its own. It is a "cholesterol absorption inhibitor" and, rather than binding bile acid, Zetia® works by blocking the absorption of intestinal cholesterol from all sources (dietary cholesterol and bile acid). The general concept is similar. Both drug classes reduce the amount of cholesterol that enters the bloodstream.

Understanding Blood Clots

You bleed after cutting or scraping your skin, but, after a few minutes, the blood hardens and the bleeding stops. This is blood clotting. Blood can also clot inside a blood vessel, and when it does, the results can be dangerous. A blood clot in the leg is called Deep Vein Thrombosis (DVT). A DVT can travel to the lungs and cause a potentially fatal event called a Pulmonary Embolism (PE). A blood clot in the heart can cause a Myocardial Infarction (MI). A blood clot that travels to the brain can cause a stroke. Naturally, you should be wondering... what exactly is a blood clot?

WHAT IS A BLOOD CLOT?

A blood clot is a clump of hard, sticky material composed of two substances – fibrin and platelets. A damaged blood vessel interacts with blood to form fibrin and to attract platelets to the site of damage. The damage can occur from a physical cut, in which case the clot forms outside of the vessel, typically on the surface of the skin. On the other hand, certain internal processes such as high blood pressure and high cholesterol can cause damage, in which case the clot forms inside the blood vessel.

PLATELETS

Platelets are a normal part of the blood. They circulate back and forth through the bloodstream along with everything else in the blood. When a blood vessel is torn, it releases chemicals that cause platelets to gather around the tear and form a plug. Then fibrin comes in and reinforces the platelet plug.

FIBRIN

Fibrin forms out of a series of chemical reactions. The reactants are liquid, and like platelets, they are a normal part of the blood. On a microscopic level, fibrin resembles little strands of fiber that form a mesh-like network around the damaged area where platelets have gathered.

THE KEY TO BLOOD CLOT PREVENTION

We can prevent blood clot formation by interfering with platelet aggregation and/or fibrin formation. Antiplatelet drugs prevent blood clot formation by interfering with platelet aggregation. Anticoagulants, on the other hand, interfere with fibrin formation.

INCREASED BLEEDING RISK

Our goal with anticoagulant and antiplatelet therapy is to prevent blood from clotting inside the blood vessels, but in doing this we also interfere with external blood clotting – the type of blood clotting that stops bleeding from cuts, scrapes, and bruises.

ANTICOAGULANTS FOR BLOOD CLOTS

BRAND NAME	GENERIC NAME
---	Heparin
Arixtra®	Fondaparinux
Coumadin®, Jantoven®	Warfarin
Eliquis®	Apixaban
Lovenox®	Enoxaparin
Pradaxa®	Dabigatran
Xarelto®	Rivaroxaban

BACKGROUND: Fibrin is one of the two major components of a blood clot. It forms out of a series of chemical reactions between blood and the chemicals released by a damaged blood vessel.

PHARMACOLOGY: Block/interfere with chemical reactions that lead to the formation of fibrin.

INDICATIONS: Prevention or Treatment of Blood Clots (e.g. Myocardial Infarction, Pulmonary Embolism, Venous Thromboembolism)

SIDE EFFECTS: Excessive Bleeding, Easy Bruising

DRUG INTERACTIONS: Foods, beverages, and supplements rich in vitamin K will interfere with the effect of warfarin. In addition, anticoagulants increase the risk of gastrointestinal bleeding when used with NSAIDs and aspirin.

BE ALERT FOR OTC NSAID AND ASPIRIN USE

Many people use an NSAID or aspirin over-the-counter for self-treating minor aches and pains. Combining these medications with an anticoagulant can lead to dangerous problems with bleeding, especially gastrointestinal bleeding. If a patient on anticoagulant therapy approaches the pharmacy counter to purchase an NSAID or aspirin, you should alert the pharmacist.

WARFARIN IS PREGNANCY CATEGORY X
NEVER TO BE USED DURING PREGNANCY

ANTIPLATELETS FOR BLOOD CLOTS

BRAND NAME	GENERIC NAME
Aggrenox®	Aspirin/Dipyridamole
Bayer Aspirin®, Ecotrin®	Aspirin
Effient®	Prasugrel
Integrilin®	Eptifibatide
Plavix®	Clopidogrel
Pletal®	Cilostazol
Reopro®	Abciximab

BACKGROUND: Platelets are one of two key components of a blood clot. They aggregate around damaged blood vessels and form a plug.

PHARMACOLOGY: Prevent/interfere with platelet aggregation.

INDICATIONS: Prevention or Treatment of Blood Clots (e.g. Myocardial Infarction, Pulmonary Embolism, Venous Thromboembolism)

SIDE EFFECTS: Excessive Bleeding, Easy Bruising

DRUG INTERACTIONS: Antiplatelet drugs increase the risk of gastrointestinal bleeding when used with NSAIDs and aspirin.

BE ALERT FOR OTC NSAID AND ASPIRIN USE

As with anticoagulants, combining OTC NSAIDs or aspirin with antiplatelet drugs can have harmful consequences. If a patient on antiplatelet therapy approaches the pharmacy counter to purchase an NSAID or aspirin, you should alert the pharmacist.

VASODILATORS FOR ANGINA

BRAND NAME	GENERIC NAME
Apresoline®	Hydralazine
Imdur®	Isosorbide Mononitrate
Isordil®	Isosorbide Dinitrate
Nitro-Bid®	Nitroglycerin (topical ointment)
Nitro-Dur®	Nitroglycerin (transdermal patch)
Nitrostat®	Nitroglycerin (sublingual tablets)

BACKGROUND: Angina is severe chest pain caused by insufficient blood flow to the heart, and it can be the precursor to a heart attack.

PHARMACOLOGY: Expand blood vessels that supply blood to the heart.

INDICATIONS: Angina, Hypertension, Heart Failure

SIDE EFFECTS: Hypotension, Headache, Dizziness

DRUG INTERACTIONS: Increased risk of hypotension when used with other medications that can lower blood pressure (especially drugs like Viagra®, Cialis®, and Levitra®).

ACUTE ANGINA TREATMENT VS ANGINA PROPHYLAXIS

There are two ways to address angina: treatment and prevention. The only option listed, above, and by far the most popular option, for treating acute angina is Nitrostat® (nitroglycerin sublingual tablets). The other drugs in the table above are for prophylaxis.

DISPENSING NITROSTAT®

The nitroglycerin in Nitrostat® is volatile, meaning it will evaporate if not stored properly. One of the storage requirements, according to the manufacturer drug package insert, is that the drug must be kept in the original glass vial at all times. For that reason, it is essential to dispense Nitrostat® in the original glass vial.

IMDUR® AND ISORDIL® ARE NOT EQUIVALENT

As their generic names suggest, Imdur® and Isordil® contain different amounts of nitrate. Imdur® (isosorbide mononitrate) contains one nitrate portion compared to the two contained in Isordil® (isosorbide dinitrate). In the body, nitrate is converted to nitric oxide, which relaxes and expands blood vessels. The mononitrate version of isosorbide is not interchangeable with the dinitrate version. It is important for pharmacy technicians to remember this when inputting prescriptions for isosorbide.

PHOSPHODIESTERASE-5 (PDE-5) INHIBITORS FOR ERECTILE DYSFUNCTION

BRAND NAME	GENERIC NAME
Viagra®	Sildenafil
Cialis®	Tadalafil
Levitra®, Staxyn®	Vardenafil

**Note: notice how the generic names of the PDE-5 Inhibitors end in "–afil."*

BACKGROUND: A common cause of erectile dysfunction (male impotence) is insufficient blood flow to the penis.

PHARMACOLOGY: Prolong the activity of nitric oxide by blocking the enzyme (PDE-5) that deactivates nitric oxide. Nitric oxide is a potent vasodilator, so it expands blood vessels and increases blood flow. Since the enzyme, PDE-5 is predominantly present in the lungs and the penis, these parts of the body are the beneficiaries of the effect. Increased blood flow to the penis leads to better, longer erections.

INDICATIONS: Erectile Dysfunction

SIDE EFFECTS: Hypotension, Priapism

DRUG INTERACTIONS: Increased risk of hypotension when used with other medications that expand blood vessels and/or lower blood pressure (especially nitroglycerin); increased risk of epistaxis (nosebleed) when used with anticoagulant or antiplatelet drugs like Coumadin® and Plavix®.

CROSS SECTION OF A BLOOD VESSEL

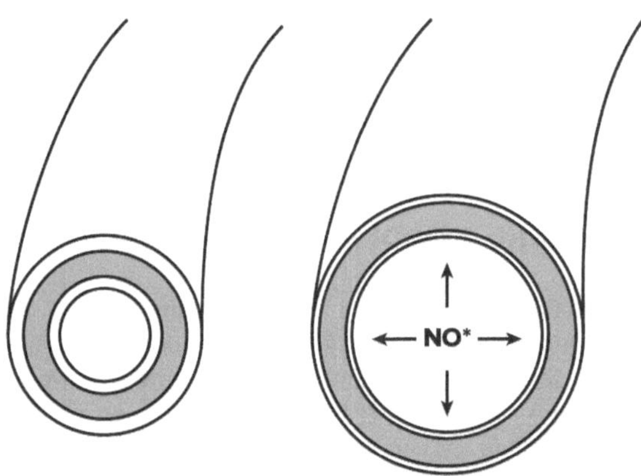

***NO = Nitric Oxide**

ANTIARRHYTHMICS
FOR CARDIAC ARRHYTHMIAS

BRAND NAME	GENERIC NAME
Pacerone®	Amiodarone
Lanoxin®	Digoxin
Norpace®	Disopyramide
Tikosyn®	Dofetilide
Tambocor®	Flecainide
Xylocaine®	Lidocaine
Rythmol®	Propafenone
Quinalan®	Quinidine

BACKGROUND: Cardiac arrhythmias are caused by irregular nerve impulses that travel through the heart.

PHARMACOLOGY: Slow down/stabilize cardiac nerve impulses.

INDICATIONS: Cardiac Arrhythmias

SIDE EFFECTS: New or Worsened Cardiac Arrhythmias

DRUG INTERACTIONS: When taken with drugs that prolong the QT interval, life-threatening cardiac arrhythmias can result.

ANTIEMETICS FOR NAUSEA AND VOMITING

BRAND NAME	GENERIC NAME	
Zofran®	Ondansetron	RX ONLY
Compazine®	Prochlorperazine	
Phenergan®	Promethazine	
Phenadoz®	Promethazine (suppository)	
Transderm-Scop®	Scopolamine (patch)	
Dramamine®	Dimenhydrinate	OTC
Antivert®, Bonine®, Dramamine® II	Meclizine	

BACKGROUND: Nausea and vomiting are associated with motion sickness, cancer chemotherapy, food poisoning, viral infections, and many other conditions and events. On a molecular level, the process is mediated by a variety of neurotransmitters, including acetylcholine, serotonin, histamine, and dopamine.

PHARMACOLOGY: There are several different classes of antiemetic drugs, each with a distinct mechanism of action, but all of those listed above work by blocking the action of one or more neurotransmitters. For example, Zofran® (Ondansetron) works by blocking the serotonin receptors that are associated with nausea and vomiting.

INDICATIONS: Nausea and Vomiting, Motion Sickness

SIDE EFFECTS: Drowsiness, Constipation

DRUG INTERACTIONS: Increased drowsiness when combined with opioids, benzodiazepines, alcohol, and/or other medications that cause drowsiness.

SELECTIVE SEROTONIN REUPTAKE INHIBITORS (SSRIs) FOR DEPRESSION

BRAND NAME	GENERIC NAME
Celexa®	Citalopram
Lexapro®	Escitalopram
Prozac®	Fluoxetine
Luvox®	Fluvoxamine
Paxil®	Paroxetine
Zoloft®	Sertraline

BACKGROUND: Serotonin (chemical name: 5-hydroxytryptamine (5-HT)) is a neurotransmitter that plays a key role in depression, behavior, eating, and nausea/vomiting. Serotonin must be available in the synaptic cleft (the open space between neurons) long enough to exert an effect. When neurons reabsorb (or "reuptake") serotonin, the serotonin is removed from the synaptic cleft and is no longer in a location where it can exert its effect.

PHARMACOLOGY: Block the reuptake of serotonin, allowing serotonin to remain in the synaptic cleft where it has more time to exert its effect.

INDICATIONS: Depression, Behavior Disorders, Eating Disorders

SIDE EFFECTS: Changes in Body Weight, Nausea, Diarrhea, Serotonin Syndrome

DRUG INTERACTIONS: Increased risk of bleeding when used with NSAIDs, anticoagulants, and/or antiplatelets. Also, increased risk of serotonin syndrome when used with other medications that increase the effect of serotonin (e.g. SNRIs, TCAs).

NOTES: All antidepressants have the potential to cause suicidal ideation and behavior in young patients – ages 24 years and under. Patients should not abruptly stop taking an SSRI without consulting their physician.

SYMPTOMS OF SEROTONIN SYNDROME

Changes in mental status (e.g. agitation, confusion, hallucinations), pressured speech, tremor*, rigidity, diarrhea, fever, sweating, flushing, and seizures.

*Tremor is the hallmark symptom of serotonin syndrome.

SEROTONIN-NOREPINEPHRINE REUPTAKE INHIBITORS (SNRIs) FOR DEPRESSION

BRAND NAME	GENERIC NAME
Pristiq®	Desvenlafaxine
Cymbalta®	Duloxetine
Savella®	Milnacipran
Effexor®	Venlafaxine

BACKGROUND: Norepinephrine also plays a role in mood and energy levels.

PHARMACOLOGY: SNRIs work just like SSRIs, but in addition to blocking the reuptake of serotonin, they also block the reuptake of norepinephrine.

INDICATIONS: Depression, Eating Disorders, Generalized Anxiety Disorder, Diabetic Peripheral Neuropathy

SIDE EFFECTS: Side effects of SNRIs are similar to those of SSRIs (e.g. serotonin syndrome), but because they increase the effect of norepinephrine, they also have cardiovascular side effects (e.g. heart palpitations, hypertension, tachycardia).

DRUG INTERACTIONS: Increased risk of serotonin syndrome when taken with other drugs that increase serotonin activity (e.g. SSRIs, TCAs).

NOTES: All antidepressants have the potential to cause suicidal ideation and behavior in young patients – ages 24 years and under. Patients should not abruptly stop taking an SNRI without consulting their physician.

TRICYCLIC ANTIDEPRESSANTS (TCAs)
FOR DEPRESSION

BRAND NAME	GENERIC NAME
Elavil®	Amitriptyline
Sinequan®	Doxepin
Pamelor®	Nortriptyline
Tofranil®	Imipramine

BACKGROUND: Serotonin and norepinephrine play a role in mood and energy levels.

PHARMACOLOGY: Block the reuptake of serotonin and norepinephrine.

INDICATIONS: Depression, Eating Disorders, Generalized Anxiety Disorder, Diabetic Peripheral Neuropathy

SIDE EFFECTS: Tachycardia, Heart Palpitations, Hypertension, Dry Mouth, Weight Gain, Reduced Sex Drive, Serotonin Syndrome

DRUG INTERACTIONS: Increased risk of serotonin syndrome when taken with other drugs that increase serotonin activity (e.g. SSRIs, SNRIs).

NOTES: Tricyclic antidepressants are an older class of antidepressants. They generally have more side effects and drug interactions. SNRIs and TCAs are also occasionally prescribed for the treatment of certain kinds of pain. All antidepressants have the potential to cause suicidal ideation and behavior in young patients – ages 24 years and under. Patients should not abruptly stop taking a TCA without consulting their physician.

DIABETES AND INSULIN

The human body is an organized collection of cells. Each cell uses glucose as the primary source of energy. Glucose is present in the blood, but cells need insulin to obtain glucose from the blood (see illustration below). In type II diabetes, the cells respond poorly to insulin and/or the pancreas fails to secrete sufficient amounts of insulin. In either case, the cells are not able to consume glucose from the blood, and glucose builds up in the bloodstream. High levels of glucose in the blood have a damaging effect on blood vessels and nerve cells. Severe damage to the blood vessels and neurons eventually leads to conditions like renal failure and blindness, which are typical of consequences of poorly managed diabetes.

TYPE I VS TYPE II DIABETES

As mentioned above, in type II diabetes, the cells respond poorly to insulin and/or the pancreas fails to secrete the amount of insulin needed to maintain normal blood glucose levels. Patients with type II diabetes do not always require insulin injections. Many patients with type II diabetes can control their blood sugar with diet, exercise, and oral antidiabetics (e.g. metformin, sulfonylureas, DPP-4 inhibitors). Type I diabetes is different. In type I diabetes, the pancreas produces such little insulin that patients with this disease are not able to survive without insulin injections. In the United States, only 1 in 20 diabetic patients have type I diabetes. Type II diabetes is much more common, mainly due to the obesity epidemic.

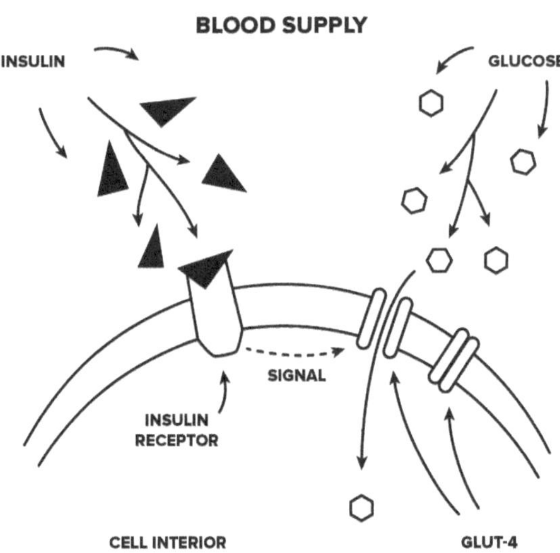

INSULIN FOR DIABETES

BRAND NAME	GENERIC NAME	
NovoLog®	Insulin Aspart	RX ONLY
Tresiba®	Insulin Degludec	
Levemir®	Insulin Detemir	
Lantus®, Toujeo®	Insulin Glargine	
Apidra®	Insulin Glulisine	
Humalog®	Insulin Lispro	
Humalog 75/25®	Mixture of 75% Lispro Protamine Insulin and 25% Lispro Insulin	
Humulin R®, Novolin R®	Regular Human Insulin	OTC
Humulin N®, Novolin N®	Insulin NPH	
Novolin 70/30®, Humulin 70/30®	Mixture of 70% Insulin NPH and 30% Regular Human Insulin	

BACKGROUND: When food enters the intestinal tract, the nutrients are absorbed into the bloodstream. The body derives glucose, a type of sugar, from carbohydrate-containing foods and uses the glucose as a source of energy.

PHARMACOLOGY: Stimulate cellular uptake of glucose from the blood. There are several different insulin formulations, each of which can be categorized based on how fast they start working (onset of action) and how long they work (duration of action).

Category	Brand Name	Onset of Action	Duration of Action
Rapid Acting	Apidra®, Humalog®, NovoLog®	15 - 30 min.	3 - 6 hours
Short Acting	Humulin R®, Novolin R®	30 - 60 min.	6 - 10 hours
Intermediate Acting	Humulin N®, Novolin N®	1 - 2 hours	16 - 24 hours
Long Acting	Lantus®, Levemir®, Toujeo®	1 - 2 hours	24 hours
Ultra Long Acting	Tresiba®	1 hour	24 - 40 hours

INDICATIONS: Type I Diabetes, Type II Diabetes

SIDE EFFECTS: Hypoglycemia, Redness/Swelling/Itching at the Injection Site

DRUG INTERACTIONS: Several drugs (e.g. thyroid hormones, diuretics, corticosteroids) can increase blood sugar, opposing the effect of insulin. Likewise, several drugs (e.g. oral antidiabetics) can decrease blood sugar, increasing the risk of hypoglycemia.

NOTES: **KEEP REFRIGERATED** until dispensed. Insulin expires after 28 days at room temperature and/or once the rubber stopper of the vial is punctured. With the exception of U-500 insulin and a certain insulin pens (e.g. Toujeo®), the concentration of all insulin is 100 units per milliliter (each 0.01 mL of liquid has 1 unit of insulin). With U-500 insulin, each milliliter contains 500 units of insulin.

REFRIGERATE
DO NOT FREEZE

BIGUANIDES FOR DIABETES

BRAND NAME	GENERIC NAME
Glucophage®, Fortamet®	Metformin

BACKGROUND: Patients with diabetes have high blood glucose levels.

PHARMACOLOGY: Lowers blood glucose levels by three mechanisms:

1. Decreases amount of glucose produced by the liver.
2. Decreases intestinal absorption of glucose.
3. Improves cellular response to insulin.

Since metformin does not increase insulin secretion, it does not cause hypoglycemia. This is one reason why metformin is so popular.

INDICATIONS: Type II Diabetes

SIDE EFFECTS: Lactic Acidosis, Vitamin B12 Deficiency, Diarrhea, Nausea/Vomiting

DRUG INTERACTIONS: Cimetidine can increase metformin levels by up to 50%.

NOTES: Metformin is one of the most commonly prescribed diabetes medications. Do not be surprised if you see a patient on metformin also getting prescriptions for vitamin B12 injections (see side effects). Diarrhea, nausea, and vomiting are common during the first few days or weeks after beginning metformin, but patients develop a tolerance over time. Prescribers will often start patients on low doses and increase to the optimal therapeutic dose over the course of a few weeks. This strategy reduces the incidence of side effects for patients that have not yet formed a tolerance to metformin. For example, the instructions may look something like this:

Metformin 500 mg

Take one tablet by mouth once daily for one week, then one tablet twice daily for one week, then two tablets twice daily thereafter

If the patient started with two tablets twice daily right off the bat, the effect on blood glucose would be better, but they would be more likely to experience diarrhea, nausea, and vomiting, and thus less likely to continue taking the medication because of the unpleasant side effects.

EXTENDED-RELEASE METFORMIN HAS FEWER SIDE EFFECTS

Extended-release versions of metformin are more expensive, but are associated with fewer side effects, particularly diarrhea, nausea, and vomiting. Some prescribers prefer to prescribe extended-release metformin for this reason.

SULFONYLUREAS FOR DIABETES

BRAND NAME	GENERIC NAME
Amaryl®	Glimepiride
Glucotrol®	Glipizide
DiaBeta®, Micronase®	Glyburide

BACKGROUND: The pancreas secretes Insulin, but in type II diabetes, the pancreas may fail to secrete sufficient amounts of insulin.

PHARMACOLOGY: Stimulate the pancreas to secrete insulin.

INDICATIONS: Type II Diabetes

SIDE EFFECTS: Hypoglycemia, Weight Gain

DRUG INTERACTIONS: Many drugs can increase the risk of hypoglycemia. Likewise, several drugs can reduce the effect of sulfonylureas.

NOTES: Another term for the sulfonylurea is "secretagogue," because they stimulate insulin secretion.

TAKE WITH FOOD

DIPEPTIDYL PEPTIDASE-4 (DPP-4) INHIBITORS FOR DIABETES

BRAND NAME	GENERIC NAME
Nesina®	Alogliptin
Tradjenta®	Linagliptin
Onglyza®	Saxagliptin
Januvia®	Sitagliptin

**Note: notice how the generic names of the DPP-4 Inhibitors end "–gliptin."*

BACKGROUND: Naturally present in the human body, incretins are hormones that signal the pancreas to increase insulin release.

PHARMACOLOGY: Delay the breakdown of incretins, thus increasing their activity. Increased incretin activity leads to increased insulin secretion.

INDICATIONS: Type II Diabetes

SIDE EFFECTS: Hypoglycemia, Muscle Pain, SJS (rare)

DRUG INTERACTIONS: Increased risk of hypoglycemia when used with other diabetes medications.

GLP-1 AGONISTS FOR DIABETES

BRAND NAME	GENERIC NAME
Byetta®, Bydureon®	Exenatide
Victoza®	Liraglutide

BACKGROUND: Incretins are hormones that are naturally produced by the body. They signal the pancreas to increase insulin release.

PHARMACOLOGY: Mimic incretins to signal the pancreas to increase insulin release.

INDICATIONS: Type II Diabetes

SIDE EFFECTS: Nausea/Vomiting, Diarrhea, Constipation

DRUG INTERACTIONS: Increased risk of hypoglycemia when used with other diabetes medications.

NOTES: Manufacturers supply GLP-1 agonists in pens for injection. It is important to **KEEP REFRIGERATED** until dispensed. According to the package inserts, Victoza® and Byetta® should be discarded after 30 days at room temperature and/or 30 days after initial use, whichever comes first. Patients should discard Bydureon® after 28 days at room temperature or 30 days after initial use, whichever comes first.

REFRIGERATE
DO NOT FREEZE

Understanding Acid Reflux

The stomach contains strong acid, and this acid has two very important functions. First, it kills bacteria, preventing infectious organisms from entering the body. Second, it begins the process of breaking down and digesting food. The stomach has mechanisms to protect itself from the corrosive effects of acid, but the esophagus does not. Acid reflux, or heartburn, occurs when acid from the stomach overflows or splashes up into the esophagus (see illustration). Most people experience heartburn on an occasional basis, usually after consuming spicy or greasy food, but other people can experience heartburn more frequently. Physicians may diagnose these individuals with a condition known as Gastroesophageal Reflux Disease (GERD). GERD is a chronic condition. Over time, the acid can severely damage the esophagus and cause serious problems.

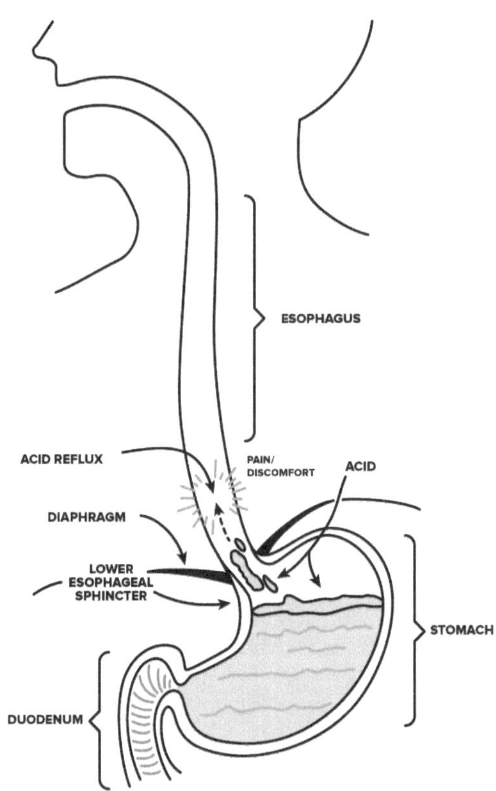

ANTACIDS FOR ACID REFLUX

BRAND NAME	GENERIC NAME	
Gaviscon®	Aluminum Hydroxide/Magnesium Carbonate	OTC
Mylanta®	Aluminum Hydroxide/Magnesium Carbonate/Simethicone	
Rolaids®	Calcium Carbonate/Magnesium Hydroxide	
Tums®, Maalox®	Calcium Carbonate	

BACKGROUND: Bases neutralize acids.

PHARMACOLOGY: Neutralize stomach acid, converting the acid to water.

INDICATIONS: Heartburn, Upset Stomach

SIDE EFFECTS: Constipation (Calcium and Aluminum), Diarrhea (Magnesium), Kidney Stones (Calcium)

DRUG INTERACTIONS: Antacids interfere with the absorption of certain medications.

ANTACID SIDE EFFECTS ACCORDING TO ELEMENTAL CONTENT

Element	Constipation	Diarrhea	Kidney Stones
Aluminum	✓		
Calcium	✓		✓
Magnesium		✓	

HISTAMINE-2 RECEPTOR ANTAGONISTS (H_2-BLOCKERS) FOR ACID REFLUX

BRAND NAME	GENERIC NAME	
Tagamet®	Cimetidine	OTC
Pepcid®	Famotidine	OTC
Axid®	Nizatidine	OTC
Zantac®	Ranitidine	OTC

**Note: notice how the generic names of the H_2-blockers end "–tidine."*

BACKGROUND: Histamine binds to H_2 receptors and increases stomach acid production.

PHARMACOLOGY: H_2–blockers prevent histamine from binding to H_2 receptors, thus preventing stomach acid production.

INDICATIONS: Heartburn, Gastroesophageal Reflux Disease (GERD)

SIDE EFFECTS: Constipation, Gynecomastia (with Cimetidine only)

DRUG INTERACTIONS: Some drugs rely on stomach acid for absorption. Since H_2 blockers reduce stomach acid, absorption of certain drugs may be impaired.

PROTON PUMP INHIBITORS (PPIs)
FOR ACID REFLUX

BRAND NAME	GENERIC NAME	
Dexilant®	Dexlansoprazole	Rx
Protonix®	Pantoprazole	Rx
Nexium®	Esomeprazole	OTC
Prevacid®	Lansoprazole	OTC
Prilosec®	Omeprazole	OTC
AciPhex®	Rabeprazole	OTC

**Note: notice how the generic names of the PPIs end "–prazole."*

BACKGROUND: Structures in the stomach known as "proton pumps" are responsible for producing acid.

PHARMACOLOGY: Proton pump inhibitors interfere with the function of proton pumps, thus decreasing the amount of acid in the stomach.

INDICATIONS: Heartburn, Gastroesophageal Reflux Disease (GERD)

SIDE EFFECTS: Abdominal Pain, Diarrhea, Nausea/Vomiting, Bone Fractures

DRUG INTERACTIONS: Omeprazole may decrease the effect of Plavix® (Clopidogrel). In addition, some drugs rely on stomach acid for optimal absorption. Since PPIs reduce stomach acid, absorption of certain drugs may be impaired.

ANTI-EPILEPTIC DRUGS (AEDs)
FOR SEIZURES

BRAND NAME		GENERIC NAME
Tegretol®, Epitol®		Carbamazepine
Depakote®		Divalproex
Neurontin®		Gabapentin
Vimpat®	C-V	Lacosamide
Lamictal®		Lamotrigine
Keppra®		Levetiracetam
Trileptal®		Oxcarbazepine
Dilantin®		Phenytoin
Lyrica®	C-V	Pregabalin
Topamax®		Topiramate
Zonegran®		Zonisamide

BACKGROUND: Seizures are caused by abnormal, hyperactive nerve function.

PHARMACOLOGY: Anti-epileptic drugs work by suppressing nerve activity. There are various mechanisms by which this is accomplished (e.g. sodium ion channel modulation, GABA* receptor stimulation, glutamate** receptor antagonism).

INDICATIONS: Seizures, Nerve Pain, Psychiatric Disorders

SIDE EFFECTS: Drowsiness, Mental Slowness, Weight Gain, Rash, SJS (rare)

DRUG INTERACTIONS: Severe nervous system suppression when combined with other drugs that suppress the nervous system (e.g. benzodiazepines, opioids, alcohol).

NOTES: Anti-epileptic drugs are also referred to as anticonvulsants.

* GABA (gamma-aminobutyric acid) is the primary *inhibitory* neurotransmitter of the central nervous system. It slows things down.

** Glutamate is the primary *excitatory* neurotransmitter of the central nervous system.

ANTIBIOTICS FOR BACTERIAL INFECTIONS

BRAND NAME	GENERIC NAME
Amoxil®	Amoxicillin
Augmentin®	Amoxicillin/Clavulanate
Unasyn®	Ampicillin/Sulbactam
Zithromax®, Z-pak®	Azithromycin
Keflex®	Cephalexin
Cipro®	Ciprofloxacin
Biaxin®	Clarithromycin
Levaquin®	Levofloxacin
Flagyl®	Metronidazole
Avelox®	Moxifloxacin
Veetids®	Penicillin
Zosyn®	Piperacillin/Tazobactam
Bactrim®, Septra®	Sulfamethoxazole/Trimethoprim
Vancocin®	Vancomycin

BACKGROUND: Bacteria are living cells. Humans are also made up of living cells, but there are several structural and physiological differences between human cells and bacterial cells.

PHARMACOLOGY: There are many different classes of antibiotics, each with a distinct mechanism of action, but every antibiotic works by exploiting a difference between bacterial cells and human cells. For instance, Clarithromycin kills living cells by binding to a structure that is only present in bacterial cells. Human cells are unaffected.

INDICATIONS: Bacterial Infections

FINISH ALL MEDICATION
UNLESS DIRECTED OTHERWISE

SIDE EFFECTS: Diarrhea

DRUG INTERACTIONS: Antibiotics increase the effect of warfarin, leading to an increased risk of bleeding. They also decrease the effect of oral contraceptives. Additionally, certain electrolytes found in antacids and multivitamins can impair antibiotic absorption.

NOTES: Unless directed otherwise by their healthcare provider, a patient should not discontinue antibiotic therapy until the entire course of treatment has been completed. When antibiotics are discontinued early, the bacteria causing the infection can develop resistance to the antibiotic. By finishing the full course of treatment, the patient increases the probability of wiping out/eradicating all of the infection-causing bacteria.

PRECAUTIONARY MEASURE TO PREVENT ALLERGIC REACTIONS

Patients commonly report allergies to penicillin and sulfa antibiotics. In some cases, those allergies are severe and life threatening. To prevent cross-contamination with medication residue, clean the counting tray and spatula with 70% isopropyl alcohol (or similar) after counting drugs like Sulfamethoxazole/Trimethoprim and Penicillin.

NON-STEROIDAL ANTI-INFLAMMATORY DRUGS (NSAIDs) FOR PAIN/INFLAMMATION

BRAND NAME	GENERIC NAME	
Celebrex®	Celecoxib	RX ONLY
Voltaren®	Diclofenac	
Indocin®	Indomethacin	
Lodine®	Etodolac	
Mobic®	Meloxicam	
Relafen®	Nabumetone	
Toradol®	Ketorolac	
Aleve®, Naprosyn®	Naproxen	OTC
Bayer Aspirin Extra Strength®	Aspirin	
Motrin®, Advil®	Ibuprofen	

BACKGROUND: Inflammation commonly causes pain. The process of inflammation is mediated by prostaglandins, which are naturally produced within the body.

PHARMACOLOGY: Block cyclooxygenase (COX), the enzyme responsible for the production of prostaglandins.

INDICATIONS: Pain, Inflammation, Fever

SIDE EFFECTS: Nausea and Vomiting, Stomach Ulcers, Renal Impairment

DRUG INTERACTIONS: Increased risk of bleeding (especially gastrointestinal bleeding) when used with anticoagulant and/or antiplatelet drugs.

NOTES: Prostaglandins also play a key role in protecting the lining of the stomach from acid-related damage. For that reason, long-term NSAID use can lead to stomach ulcers. Also worth noting, aspirin is a little different from the other NSAIDs. Aspirin not only has anti-inflammatory effects, but also antiplatelet effects (i.e. aspirin helps prevent blood clot formation). For that reason, practitioners often prescribe aspirin for heart attack and stroke prevention. As a side note, NSAIDs commonly cause nausea and upset stomach. To prevent these side effects, we often recommend taking NSAIDs with food.

TAKE WITH FOOD

OPIOIDS FOR PAIN

BRAND NAME		GENERIC NAME
various combination products*	C-III – C-V	Codeine
various combination products**	C-II	Hydrocodone
Dilaudid®	C-II	Hydromorphone
MS Contin®, Kadian®	C-II	Morphine (extended-release)
Roxanol®	C-II	Morphine (immediate-release)
Oxycontin®	C-II	Oxycodone (extended-release)
Roxicodone®	C-II	Oxycodone (immediate-release)
Ultram®	C-IV	Tramadol

* Robitussin® AC, Tylenol® #3

** Norco®, Lortab®, Vicodin®, Tussionex®, Tussigon®

BACKGROUND: Activation of opioid receptors produces analgesia and sedation.

PHARMACOLOGY: Activate opioid receptors, providing pain relief.

INDICATIONS: Pain, Cough

SIDE EFFECTS: Sedation, Respiratory Depression, Constipation, Dependency

DRUG INTERACTIONS: Increased incidence of sedation and respiratory depression when taken with other drugs that suppress the nervous system (e.g. benzodiazepines, alcohol).

NOTES: All of the opioid analgesics are controlled substances. For patients that have used an opioid on a long-term basis, the opioid must be discontinued gradually over time to avoid withdrawal symptoms. Constipation is the only side effect to which patients do not develop a tolerance when using opioids on a long-term basis. Also worth noting, codeine by itself (when not present in combination with another drug) is a Schedule II controlled substance.

MAY CAUSE DROWSINESS

BENZODIAZEPINES FOR ANXIETY

BRAND NAME		GENERIC NAME
Xanax®	C-IV	Alprazolam
Librium®	C-IV	Chlordiazepoxide
Onfi®	C-IV	Clobazam
Klonopin®	C-IV	Clonazepam
Valium®, Diastat®	C-IV	Diazepam
Ativan®	C-IV	Lorazepam
Versed®	C-IV	Midazolam
Restoril®	C-IV	Temazepam
Halcion®	C-IV	Triazolam

**Note: notice how the generic names of most of the benzodiazepines end in "–azepam" or "-azolam."*

BACKGROUND: There are two types of benzodiazepine receptors – BNZ_1 and BNZ_2. BNZ_1 receptor activation promotes sleep and BNZ_2 receptor activation promotes muscle relaxation.

PHARMACOLOGY: Benzodiazepines bind to benzodiazepine receptors (BNZ_1 and BNZ_2) and enhance the effect of GABA (gamma-aminobutyric acid; the primary inhibitory neurotransmitter of the central nervous system). These effects are useful in the treatment of anxiety, insomnia, muscle spasms, and other conditions.

INDICATIONS: Anxiety, Insomnia, Agitation, Seizures, Muscle Spasms, Alcohol Withdrawal

SIDE EFFECTS: Drowsiness, Somnolence, Dependency

DRUG INTERACTIONS: Increased drowsiness when used with other drugs that suppress the nervous system (e.g. sedative-hypnotics, opioids, anticonvulsants, alcohol).

NOTES: All drugs in this class are Schedule IV controlled substances according to federal law (individual state laws may be more stringent).

MAY CAUSE DROWSINESS

SEDATIVE-HYPNOTICS FOR INSOMNIA

BRAND NAME		GENERIC NAME
Lunesta®	C-IV	Eszopiclone
Sonata®	C-IV	Zaleplon
Ambien®	C-IV	Zolpidem

BACKGROUND: BNZ_1 receptor activation promotes sleep.

PHARMACOLOGY: Bind to BNZ_1 receptors, promoting sleep.

INDICATIONS: Insomnia

SIDE EFFECTS: Drowsiness, Somnolence, Dependency

DRUG INTERACTIONS: Increased drowsiness when used with other drugs that suppress nervous system activity (e.g. benzodiazepines, opioids, antihistamines, alcohol).

NOTES: All drugs in this class are Schedule IV controlled substances.

MAY CAUSE DROWSINESS

STIMULANTS FOR ADHD

BRAND NAME		GENERIC NAME
Adderall®	C-II	Amphetamine/Dextroamphetamine
Strattera®		Atomoxetine
Kapvay®		Clonidine
Focalin®	C-II	Dexmethylphenidate
Intuniv®		Guanfacine
Vyvanse®	C-II	Lisdexamfetamine
Daytrana®	C-II	Methylphenidate (patch)
Ritalin®	C-II	Methylphenidate
Concerta®	C-II	Methylphenidate (extended-release)

BACKGROUND: A major symptom of Attention Deficit Hyperactivity Disorder (ADHD) is poor mental focus.

PHARMACOLOGY: Stimulate the central nervous system (i.e. the brain), thereby improving mental focus.

INDICATIONS: ADHD, Narcolepsy

SIDE EFFECTS: Insomnia, Hypertension, Dependency

DRUG INTERACTIONS: Use with other stimulants, such as caffeine and weight-loss drugs, increases the risk of high blood pressure and cardiovascular problems.

Understanding Asthma and COPD

LUNG DISEASE AND CONSTRICTED AIRWAYS

Asthma and Chronic Obstructive Pulmonary Disease (COPD) are characterized by poor lung function and difficulty breathing. One of the primary ways we can treat these diseases is with drugs that expand/dilate the airways, making it easier for patients to breathe. There are two types of receptors relevant to this conversation: beta-receptors, activation of which stimulates airway dilation, and acetylcholine receptors, activation of which stimulates airway constriction.

BETA-RECEPTORS

Substances such as epinephrine and norepinephrine activate beta-receptors. In the airways, activation of these receptors leads to airway expansion/dilation. For lung diseases such as asthma and COPD, this effect can be very therapeutic. Consequently, many asthma and COPD drugs are beta-receptor agonists.

ACETYLCHOLINE RECEPTORS

In the lungs, acetylcholine receptor activation causes the airways to constrict. This makes breathing difficult for patients with lung disease. For that reason, we use drugs that block or prevent the activation of acetylcholine receptors. These are called acetylcholine receptor antagonists, or "anticholinergics."

INFLAMMATION

Besides airway constriction, inflammation is also associated with asthma and COPD. For that reason, practitioners frequently prescribe inhaled corticosteroids to suppress airway inflammation in these patients.

THE USE OF INHALED DOSAGE FORMS

Most of the drugs used to treat asthma and COPD are manufactured as inhaled dosage forms, such as nebulizer solutions, metered dose inhalers, and dry powder inhalers. These dosage forms allow the medication to be delivered directly to the site of action inside the lungs. When a drug is taken systemically (e.g. orally or by injection), it enters the blood stream and travels to all areas of the body, which can cause many side effects. When a drug is applied locally, directly to the site of action, as is the case with inhaled dosage forms in the treatment of lung disease, this not only maximizes the effectiveness of the medication, but also minimizes side effects because it prevents other areas of the body from being exposed to the drug.

INHALED BETA AGONISTS
FOR ASTHMA AND COPD

BRAND NAME	GENERIC NAME	
ProAir®, Proventil®, Ventolin® HFA	Albuterol (inhaler)	SHORT ACTING
AccuNeb®	Albuterol (nebulizer solution)	
Xopenex® HFA	Levalbuterol (inhaler)	
Xopenex®	Levalbuterol (nebulizer solution)	
Brovana®	Arformoterol (nebulizer solution)	LONG ACTING
Foradil Aerolizer®	Formoterol (inhaler)	
Perforomist®	Formoterol (inhaler)	
Serevent®	Salmeterol (diskus/inhaler)	

BACKGROUND: One of the main problems in asthma and COPD is narrowed airways. When beta-receptors in the lungs are activated, the airways dilate.

PHARMACOLOGY: Activate beta-receptors in the lungs to dilate the airways, making it easier for patients to breathe.

INDICATIONS: Asthma, COPD

SIDE EFFECTS: Tachycardia, Palpitations

DRUG INTERACTIONS: Certain beta-blockers (e.g. carvedilol) can oppose the effect of inhaled beta agonists.

NOTES: There are two classes of inhaled beta agonists – short acting and long acting. Patients normally use the short acting beta agonists for asthma attacks, thus the term "rescue inhaler" is used for albuterol inhalers. The typical asthma patient only uses short acting beta agonists on an "as needed" basis, not on a schedule. On the other hand, prescribers employ long acting beta agonists to prevent symptoms of asthma or COPD. Long acting beta agonists are not effective for acute asthma attacks, and they are used on a scheduled daily basis.

FOR INHALATION ONLY

INHALED ANTICHOLINERGICS
FOR ASTHMA AND COPD

BRAND NAME	GENERIC NAME
Atrovent®	Ipratropium (nebulizer solution)
Atrovent® HFA	Ipratropium (inhaler)
Spiriva® Respimat	Tiotropium (inhaler)
Spriva® HandiHaler	Tiotropium (capsules for inhalation)

BACKGROUND: As with asthma, one of the main problems in COPD is narrowed airways. Activation of acetylcholine receptors in the lungs leads to airway constriction/narrowing.

PHARMACOLOGY: Block activation of acetylcholine receptors, thereby reducing airway constriction.

INDICATIONS: COPD

SIDE EFFECTS: Dry Mouth, Constipation

DRUG INTERACTIONS: For patients experiencing constipation from opioid uses, the addition of an inhaled anticholinergic drug can worsen this constipation.

NOTES: Ipratropium is a short acting anticholinergic inhaled four times daily, whereas tiotropium is long acting and is inhaled once daily. Anticholinergics are not effective for the treatment of acute asthma symptoms ("asthma attacks").

FOR INHALATION ONLY

COMBINED ANTICHOLINERGICS AND SHORT-ACTING BETA AGONISTS

Since the inhaled beta agonists and inhaled anticholinergics have a different mechanism of action, practitioners commonly prescribe both drugs for simultaneous use. For that reason, manufacturers developed a combination albuterol and ipratropium inhaler and nebulizer solution (see below).

BRAND NAME	GENERIC NAME
Combivent Respimat®	Ipratropium/Albuterol (inhaler)
DuoNeb®	Ipratropium/Albuterol (nebulizer solution)

INHALED CORTICOSTEROIDS
FOR ASTHMA AND COPD

BRAND NAME	GENERIC NAME
Asmanex®	Mometasone
Flovent®	Fluticasone
Pulmicort®	Budesonide
Qvar®	Beclomethasone

BACKGROUND: Inflammation plays a major role in asthma and COPD.

PHARMACOLOGY: Block the body's natural mechanism for production of inflammatory mediators, thus reducing inflammation.

INDICATIONS: Asthma, COPD

SIDE EFFECTS: Oral Thrush, Upper Respiratory Infection

DRUG INTERACTIONS: Certain drugs can increase or decrease the activity of corticosteroids.

NOTES: For inhaled corticosteroid prescriptions, many practitioners include the instructions: "rinse mouth after use." This is because corticosteroid residue left in the mouth can cause oral thrush, a fungal infection in the mouth.

RINSE MOUTH AFTER USE

COMBINED CORTICOSTEROIDS AND LONG-ACTING BETA AGONISTS

Many inhaled corticosteroids are available in combination with long acting beta agonists for prevention of severe symptoms in patients with asthma or COPD. Since they are preventative, patients use these drugs on a scheduled daily basis – usually one or two inhalations twice daily. Examples are listed below.

BRAND NAME	GENERIC NAME
Advair®	Fluticasone/Salmeterol
Dulera®	Mometasone/Formoterol
Symbicort®	Budesonide/Formoterol

MUSCLE RELAXANTS FOR MUSCLE SPASMS

BRAND NAME		GENERIC NAME
Lioresal®		Baclofen
Soma®	C-IV	Carisoprodol
Flexeril®		Cyclobenzaprine
Skelaxin®		Metaxalone
Robaxin®		Methocarbamol
Zanaflex®		Tizanidine

BACKGROUND: The nervous system mediates muscle contraction.

PHARMACOLOGY: Interfere with the nerve signals that mediate muscle contraction.

INDICATIONS: Muscle Spasm, Pulled Muscle, Back Pain

SIDE EFFECTS: Drowsiness

DRUG INTERACTIONS: Increased drowsiness/sedation when combined with other drugs that suppress nervous system activity (e.g. benzodiazepines, opioids, antihistamines, alcohol).

MAY CAUSE DROWSINESS

HORMONE CONTRACEPTIVES
FOR PREGNANCY PREVENTION

BRAND NAME	GENERIC NAME	DOSAGE FORM/ PACKAGE CONTENTS
Ortho Cyclen®	Sprintec®	21 Active & 7 Inactive Tablets
Ortho Tri-Cyclen®	Tri-Sprintec®	21 Active & 7 Inactive Tablets
Yaz®	Gianvi®	24 Active & 4 Inactive Tablets
Loestrin® 24 Fe	Lomedia® 24 Fe	24 Active & 4 Iron Tablets
Ortho Evra®	Xulane®	Transdermal Patch
NuvaRing®	*	Intravaginal ring
Depo-Provera®	Medroxyprogesterone	Intramuscular Injection
Plan B One-Step®	Next Choice One Dose®	1 Emergency Contraceptive Tablet

*No generics currently available

BACKGROUND: Normally, female hormones rise and fall in a pattern or "cycle" that promotes ovulation and implantation of an egg. During ovulation, the egg is released from the ovary. For an egg to be susceptible to fertilization by a sperm cell, ovulation must occur. Once fertilized, the egg needs to implant into the wall of the uterus to survive. If all three of these steps occur successfully – ovulation, fertilization and implantation – then pregnancy occurs.

PHARMACOLOGY: Prevent ovulation and/or implantation of the egg.

INDICATIONS: Pregnancy Prevention

DO NOT USE IF YOU ARE PREGNANT

SIDE EFFECTS: Nausea and Vomiting, Abdominal Pain, Emotional Changes, Blood Clots

DRUG INTERACTIONS: Smoking cigarettes increases the risk of blood clot formation. Antibiotics can reduce the effectiveness of hormone contraceptives.

Keep it Simple

There are dozens of hormone contraceptive products. Most of them contain an estrogen and a progestin component. The names of the active ingredients can be long and complicated. Examples include norgestrel, norgestimate, levonorgestrel, desogestrel, norethindrone, and ethinyl estradiol. To reduce confusion, many generic manufacturers sell the generic versions under a brand name. For example, Ortho Cyclen® is generically available as Sprintec® & MonoNessa®, and Ortho Tri-Cyclen® is generically available as Tri-Sprintec® & TriNessa®. This is just the tip of the iceberg. Do not be overwhelmed by all of these names. To make this subject easier to digest, the list above includes only the names of the most popular products along with details on how they are supplied/administered.

ALL HORMONE CONTRACEPTIVES ARE PREGNANCY CATEGORY X NEVER TO BE USED DURING PREGNANCY

ANTI-GOUT AGENTS FOR GOUT

BRAND NAME	GENERIC NAME
Zyloprim®	Allopurinol
Colcrys®	Colchicine
Uloric®	Febuxostat

BACKGROUND: Gout is essentially severe inflammation of one or more joints caused by high uric acid levels in the blood. Uric acid enters the blood after consuming certain foods and beverages and when cells die inside the body. Certain drugs can also increase uric acid levels. When the concentration of uric acid in the blood gets too high, it crystallizes (i.e. turns to a solid), and the uric acid crystals deposit in joint spaces. The immune system attacks the uric acid crystals, thinking they are foreign invaders. The joints suffer collateral damage from the immune response, causing severe joint pain and inflammation (i.e. gout). The joint of the big toe is usually the first to be affected.

PHARMACOLOGY: Block the formation of uric acid (Allopurinol and Febuxostat), or prevent the immune system from attacking uric acid crystals (Colchicine).

INDICATIONS: Gout

SIDE EFFECTS: Diarrhea, Nausea and Vomiting, Abdominal Cramps/Pain, Impaired White Blood Cell Formation/Development (Colchicine)

DRUG INTERACTIONS: Many drugs can increase uric acid levels in the blood (e.g. aspirin and thiazide diuretics), which can work against uric acid lowering treatments.

GOUT AND NSAIDs

During a gout flare, practitioners often prescribe an NSAID to reduce joint pain and inflammation. Indocin® (Indomethacin) is the most common NSAID used for this purpose.

OPHTHALMIC PROSTAGLANDIN ANALOGS
FOR GLAUCOMA

BRAND NAME	GENERIC NAME
Lumigan®	Bimatoprost
Xalatan®	Latanoprost
Travatan®	Travoprost

**Note: Notice that all of the generic names for prostaglandin analogs end in "-oprost."*

BACKGROUND: The front of the eye is filled with a fluid called aqueous humor. Aqueous humor normally flows into and out of the eye in equal proportions, maintaining even pressure within the eye. In patients with glaucoma, there are problems, usually with the outflow of aqueous humor, that lead to elevated pressure within the eye. Over time, this high intraocular pressure damages the optic nerve. Minor vision loss is common, and if left untreated, the vision loss will eventually progress to complete blindness.

PHARMACOLOGY: Increase the outflow of aqueous humor, thus decreasing pressure within the eye. Prostaglandins are typically associated with inflammation, but in the eye, prostaglandins increase the outflow of aqueous humor.

INDICATIONS: Glaucoma

SIDE EFFECTS: Eyelash Growth, Dry Eye, Blurred Vision, Discoloration of the Iris, Inflammation of the Eye

DRUG INTERACTIONS: None

NOTES: The medications in this drug class are eye drops. Xalatan® (Latanoprost) should be stored in the refrigerator until opened. Once opened, Xalatan® can be stored at room temperature for up to 6 weeks, after which any remaining medication must be discarded. Lumigan® and Travatan® are stable at room temperature.

FOR THE EYE

CAPITALIZING ON A SIDE EFFECT

Eyelash growth is common side effect associated with the use of prostaglandin analogs. The side effect is so common that the drug manufacturer Allergen, Inc. reformulated bimatoprost to make another prescription-only product called Latisse®, designed specifically for cosmetic eyelash enhancement.

OPHTHALMIC BETA-BLOCKERS
FOR GLAUCOMA

BRAND NAME	GENERIC NAME
Timoptic®	Timolol
Betoptic S®	Betaxolol

**Note: Notice that the generic names for beta-blockers end in "-olol."*

BACKGROUND: Aqueous humor production also contributes to high intraocular pressure.

PHARMACOLOGY: Reduce the production of aqueous humor.

INDICATIONS: Glaucoma

SIDE EFFECTS: Bradycardia, Hypotension, Asthma and COPD Exacerbations

DRUG INTERACTIONS: May increase risk of hypotension and bradycardia when used with other drugs that can lower blood pressure and reduce heart rate.

NOTES: We covered beta-blockers before in the high blood pressure section, but the beta-blockers listed here are supplied as eye drops created specifically for the treatment of glaucoma.

FOR THE EYE

PROCEED TO THE NEXT SECTION TO MEMORIZE THE TOP 200 PRESCRIPTION DRUGS

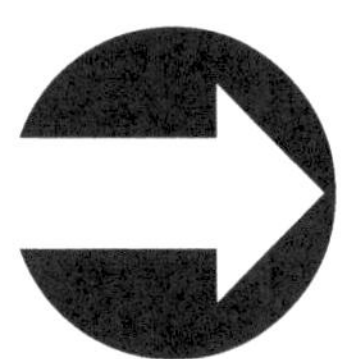

TOP 200 PRESCRIPTION DRUGS

BRAND NAME	GENERIC NAME	PRIMARY INDICATION(S)
Abilify	Aripiprazole	Psychiatric Disorders
Accupril	Quinapril	Hypertension
Aciphex	Rabeprazole	GERD
Actonel	Risedronate	Osteoporosis
Actos	Pioglitazone	Diabetes
Adderall	Amphetamine/D-Amphetamine ***C-II***	ADHD
Adipex-P	Phentermine ***C-IV***	Weight Loss
Advair	Fluticasone/Salmeterol	Asthma, COPD
Aldactone	Spironolactone	Hypertension
Allegra	Fexofenadine	Allergies
Altace	Ramipril	Hypertension
Amaryl	Glimepiride	Diabetes
Ambien	Zolpidem ***C-IV***	Insomnia
Amoxil	Amoxicillin	Bacterial Infections
Antivert	Meclizine	Motion Sickness, Vertigo
Apresoline	Hydralazine	Angina
Aricept	Donepezil	Alzheimer's Disease
Atarax	Hydroxyzine	Allergies
Ativan	Lorazepam ***C-IV***	Anxiety
AtroPen	Atropine	Cardiac Arrest
Atrovent	Ipratropium	COPD
Augmentin	Amoxicillin/Clavulanate	Bacterial Infections
Avalide	Irbesartan/Hydrochlorothiazide	Hypertension
Avandia	Rosiglitazone	Diabetes
Avapro	Irbesartan	Hypertension
Avelox	Moxifloxacin	Bacterial Infections
Bactrim, Septra	Sulfamethoxazole/Trimethoprim	Bacterial Infections
Benadryl	Diphenhydramine	Allergies
Benicar	Olmesartan	Hypertension
Biaxin	Clarithromycin	Bacterial Infections
Boniva	Ibandronate	Osteoporosis
Buspar	Buspirone	Anxiety
Byetta	Exenatide	Diabetes
Cardizem, Tiazac	Diltiazem	Hypertension, Arrhythmias
Catapress	Clonidine	Hypertension
Celebrex	Celecoxib	Inflammation, Arthritis
Celexa	Citalopram	Depression
Cheratussin AC	Guafenesin/Codeine ***C-V***	Cough

Cheratussin DAC	Guafenesin/Codeine/Pseudoephedrine *C-V*	Cough/Congestion
Cialis	Tadalafil	Erectile Dysfunction
Cipro	Ciprofloxacin	Bacterial Infections
Claritin	Loratadine	Allergies
Cleocin	Clindamycin	Bacterial Infections
Colcrys	Colchicine	Gout
Compazine	Prochlorperazine	Nausea and Vomiting
Concerta	Methylphenidate ER *C-II*	ADHD
Coreg	Carvedilol	Hypertension
Coumadin, Jantoven	Warfarin	Blood Clots
Cozaar	Losartan	Hypertension
Crestor	Rosuvastatin	High Cholesterol
Cymbalta	Duloxetine	Depression
Deltasone	Prednisone	Inflammation
Demerol	Meperidine *C-II*	Pain
Depakote	Divalproex	Seizures
Depo-Provera	Medroxyprogesterone	Birth Control
Desyrel	Trazodone	Depression, Insomnia
Detrol	Tolterodine	Overactive Bladder
Dexilant	Dexlansoprazole	GERD
Diflucan	Fluconazole	Fungal Infections
Dilantin	Phenytoin	Seizures
Dilaudid	Hydromorphone *C-II*	Pain
Diovan	Valsartan	Hypertension
Ditropan	Oxybutynin	Overactive Bladder
Duragesic	Fentanyl *C-II*	Pain
Ecotrin	Aspirin	Blood Clot Prevention, Pain
Effexor	Venlafaxine	Depression
Elavil	Amitriptyline	Depression
Ery-tab	Erythromycin	Bacterial Infections
Estrace, Evamist	Estradiol	Menopause Symptoms
Fioricet	Butalbital/Acetaminophen/Caffeine	Migraine Headaches
Flagyl	Metronidazole	Bacterial Infections
Flexeril	Cyclobenzaprine	Muscle Spasms
Flomax	Tamsulosin	Benign Prostatic Hyperplasia
Fosamax	Alendronate	Osteoporosis
Glucophage	Metformin	Diabetes
Glucotrol	Glipizide	Diabetes
Haldol	Haloperidol	Psychiatric Disorders
Humulin R, Novolin R	Regular Human Insulin	Diabetes
Hycodan, Hydromet	Hydrocodone/Homatropine *C-II*	Cough

Hytrin	Terazosin	Benign Prostatic Hyperplasia
Hyzaar	Losartan/Hydrochlorothiazide	Hypertension
Imdur	Isosorbide Mononitrate	Angina
Imitrex	Sumatriptan	Migraine Headaches
Inderal	Propranolol	Hypertension, Arrhythmias
Indocin	Indomethacin	Inflammation, Gout Flares
Isoptin, Calan	Verapamil	Hypertension, Arrhythmias
Januvia	Sitagliptin	Diabetes
Keflex	Cephalexin	Bacterial Infections
Kenalog	Triamcinolone	Inflammation, Skin Disorders
Keppra	Levetiracetam	Seizures
Klonopin	Clonazepam ***C-IV***	Anxiety
Klor-Con, K-Dur	Potassium Chloride	Hypokalemia
Lamictal	Lamotrigine	Seizures
Lanoxin	Digoxin	Cardiac Arrhythmias
Lantus	Insulin Glargine	Diabetes
Lasix	Furosemide	Hypertension, Edema
Levaquin	Levofloxacin	Bacterial Infections
Levitra, Staxyn	Vardenafil	Erectile Dysfunction
Lexapro	Escitalopram	Depression
Liorisal	Baclofen	Muscle Spasms
Lipitor	Atorvastatin	High Cholesterol
Lithobid	Lithium Carbonate	Psychiatric Disorders
Lodine	Etodolac	Inflammation
Lopressor	Metoprolol Tartrate (IR)	Hypertension, Arrhythmias
Lotrel	Amlodipine/Benazepril	Hypertension
Lovenox	Enoxaparin	Blood Clots
Lunesta	Eszopiclone ***C-IV***	Insomnia
Lyrica	Pregabalin ***C-V***	Seizures, Pain, Fibromyalgia
Maxzide, Dyazide	Hydrochlorothiazide/Triamterene	Hypertension
Medrol	Methylprednisolone	Inflammation
Methadose, Dolophine	Methadone ***C-II***	Pain
Mevacor	Lovastatin	High Cholesterol
Microzide	Hydrochlorothiazide	Hypertension
Mobic	Meloxicam	Inflammation
Motrin	Ibuprofen	Inflammation
MS Contin	Morphine Sulfate ER ***C-II***	Pain
Namenda	Memantine	Alzheimer's Disease
Naprosyn	Naproxen	Inflammation
Nasonex	Mometasone	Inflammation, Allergies
Neurontin	Gabapentin	Seizures, Nerve Pain

Nexium	Esomeprazole	GERD
Niaspan	Niacin	High Cholesterol
Nifediac, Procardia	Nifedipine	Hypertension
Nitro-Bid	Nitroglycerin Transdermal Ointment	Angina
Nitro-Dur	Nitroglycerin Transdermal Patch	Angina
Nitrostat	Nitroglycerin Sublingual Tablets	Angina
Norvasc	Amlodipine	Hypertension
Nystop	Nystatin	Fungal Infections
Omnicef	Cefdinir	Bacterial Infections
Ortho Tri-Cyclen	Ethinyl Estradiol/Norgestimate	Birth Control
Oxycontin	Oxycodone ER ***C-II***	Pain
Pacerone	Amiodarone	Cardiac Arrhythmias
Paxil	Paroxetine	Depression
Pepcid	Famotidine	GERD
Percocet, Endocet	Oxycodone/Acetaminophen ***C-II***	Pain
Phenergan	Promethazine	Nausea and Vomiting
Plavix	Clopidogrel	Blood Clots
Pravachol	Pravastatin	High Cholesterol
Premarin	Conjugated Estrogens	Menopause Symptoms
Prevacid	Lansoprazole	GERD
Prilosec	Omeprazole	GERD
Prinivil, Zestril	Lisinopril	Hypertension
Protonix	Pantoprazole	GERD
Proventil, ProAir, Ventolin	Albuterol HFA Inhaler	Asthma
Provera	Medroxyprogesterone	Irregular Menstrual Bleeding
Provigil	Modafinil ***C-IV***	Narcolepsy, Fatigue
Prozac	Fluoxetine	Depression
Reglan	Metoclopramide	GERD
Relafen	Nabumetone	Inflammation
Remeron	Mirtazapine	Depression
Requip	Ropinirole	Parkinson's Disease
Restoril	Temazepam ***C-IV***	Insomnia
Risperdal	Risperidone	Psychiatric Disorders
Ritalin	Methylphenidate ***C-II***	ADHD
Robaxin	Methocarbamol	Muscle Spasms
Roxicodone	Oxycodone ***C-II***	Pain
Seroquel	Quetiapine	Psychiatric Disorders
Sinemet	Carbidopa/Levodopa	Parkinson's Disease
Singulair	Montelukast	Asthma
Skelaxin	Metaxalone	Muscle Spasms
Soma	Carisoprodal ***C-IV***	Muscle Spasms

Spiriva	Tiotropium Inhaler	COPD
Strattera	Atomoxetine	ADHD
Synthroid	Levothyroxine	Hypothyroidism
Tamiflu	Oseltamivir	Viral Infections
Tegretol	Carbamazepine	Seizures
Tenormin	Atenolol	Hypertension, Arrhythmias
Tessalon	Benzonatate	Cough
Topamax	Topiramate	Seizures
Toprol XL	Metoprolol Succinate (ER)	Hypertension, Arrhythmias
Toradol	Ketorolac	Inflammation
Trexall	Methotrexate	Inflammation
Tricor	Fenofibrate	High Cholesterol
Tussionex	Hydrocodone/Chlorpheniramine ***C-II***	Cough
Tylenol #3	Acetaminophen/Codeine ***C-III***	Pain, Cough
Ultracet	Tramadol/Acetaminophen ***C-IV***	Pain
Ultram	Tramadol ***C-IV***	Pain
Vagifem	Estradiol	Menopause Symptoms
Valium	Diazepam ***C-IV***	Anxiety, Muscle Spasms
Valtrex	Valacyclovir	Viral Infections
Vancocin	Vancomycin	Bacterial Infections
Vasotec	Enalapril	Hypertension
Vesicare	Solifenacin	Overactive Bladder
Viagra	Sildenafil	Erectile Dysfunction
Vibramycin, Monodox	Doxycycline	Bacterial Infections
Vicodin, Norco	Hydrocodone/Acetaminophen ***C-II***	Pain
Voltaren	Diclofenac	Inflammation
Vytorin	Ezetemibe/Simvastatin	High Cholesterol
Wellbutrin XL	Bupropion (ER)	Depression
Xanax	Alprazolam ***C-IV***	Anxiety
Xilocaine, Lidoderm	Lidocaine	Arrhythmias, Pain
Zanaflex	Tizanidine	Muscle Spasms
Zantac	Ranitidine	GERD
Zetia	Ezetimibe	High Cholesterol
Zithromax, Z-Pak	Azithromycin	Bacterial Infections
Zocor	Simvastatin	High Cholesterol
Zofran	Ondansetron	Nausea and Vomiting
Zoloft	Sertraline	Depression
Zyloprim	Allopurinol	Gout
Zyrtec	Cetirizine	Allergies

TOP 45 OTC DRUGS

Over-the-counter (OTC) medications are drugs that are available to patients without a prescription for self-treatment of minor medical conditions. Below is a list of the Top 45 OTC Medications categorized by their primary uses.

OTC Pain Medications (Analgesics)

BRAND NAME	GENERIC NAME	OTHER USES
Advil®, Motrin®	Ibuprofen	Fever, Inflammation
Aleve®	Naproxen	Fever, Inflammation
Azo®	Phenazopyridine	*Urinary Pain Only
Ecotrin®	Aspirin	Fever, Blood Clot Prevention
Excedrin® Migraine	Acetaminophen/Aspirin/Caffeine	Migraine Headaches
Tylenol®	Acetaminophen	Fever

*Azo® (Phenazopyridine) is only effective for urinary pain/burning.

OTC Antacids

BRAND NAME	GENERIC NAME
Alka-Seltzer®	Citric Acid/Sodium Bicarbonate
Gaviscon®	Aluminum Hydroxide/Magnesium Carbonate
Maalox®	Aluminum Hydroxide/Magnesium Hydroxide/Simethicone
Mylanta®	Aluminum Hydroxide/Magnesium Hydroxide/Simethicone
Nexium®	Esomeprazole
Pepcid®	Famotidine
Pepto-Bismol®	Bismuth Subsalicylate
Prevacid®	Lansoprazole
Prilosec OTC®	Omeprazole
Rolaids®	Calcium Carbonate/Magnesium Hydroxide
Tagamet®	Cimetidine
Tums®	Calcium Carbonate
Zantac®	Ranitidine

*Most antacids are effective for treating heartburn, indigestion, nausea, and upset stomach. Antacids that contain aluminum or calcium are preferred for patients with diarrhea, and antacids with simethicone are good for reducing gas and bloating.

OTC Laxatives

BRAND NAME	GENERIC NAME
Citrate of Magnesium	Magnesium Citrate
Colace®	Docusate
Dulcolax®	Bisacodyl
Metamucil®	Psyllium Fiber
Milk of Magnesia®	Magnesium Hydroxide
Miralax®	Polyethylene Glycol (PEG) 3350
Senokot®	Sennosides
Senokot-S®	Docusate/Sennosides

*Laxatives are effective for treating constipation.

OTC Cough & Cold Medications

BRAND NAME	GENERIC NAME	SPECIFIC USE
Afrin® Nasal Spray	Oxymetazoline	Nasal Decongestant
Delsym®	Dextromethorphan	Cough Suppressant
Neo-Synephrine® Nasal Spray	Phenylephrine	Nasal Decongestant
Robitussin®	Guaifenesin	Expectorant
Sudafed®	Pseudoephedrine	Decongestant

OTC Allergy Medications (Antihistamines)

BRAND NAME	GENERIC NAME
Allegra®	Fexofenadine
Benadryl®	Diphenhydramine
Chlor-Trimeton®	Chlorpheniramine
Claritin®, Alavert®	Loratadine
Flonase® Nasal Spray	Fluticasone
Nasacort® Nasal Spray	Triamcinolone
Zaditor®, Alaway® Eye Drops	Ketotifen
Zyrtec®	Cetirizine

OTC Antifungals

BRAND NAME	GENERIC NAME
Lamisil®	Terbinafine
Lamisil® AF	Tolnaftate
Lotrimin®	Clotrimazole
Monistat® Vaginal Cream	Miconazole
Zeasorb®	Miconazole

*OTC antifungals are effective for treating minor topical fungal infections (e.g. jock itch, athlete's foot, and ringworm).

DRUG-DRUG INTERACTIONS

Warfarin **and** NSAIDs*

Warfarin is an anticoagulant used to prevent or treat blood clots. A major side effect of warfarin is bleeding. NSAIDs are notorious for damaging the lining of the stomach, which has the potential to lead to a gastrointestinal bleed. When warfarin and NSAIDs are used together, the risk of a life-threatening GI bleed increases significantly. NSAIDs also have some "anti-platelet" (blood-thinning) effect, which further increases bleed risk. *Some examples of generic NSAIDs include: Ibuprofen, Naproxen, Aspirin, Meloxicam, Indomethacin, and Diclofenac.

Warfarin **and** Antibiotics

Antibiotics increase the bleeding risk associated with warfarin. The reason for this is explained below.

How Warfarin Works

The body uses Vitamin K to activate the "vitamin K-dependent clotting factors" (factors 2, 7, 9, and 10). Once vitamin K is used to activate a clotting factor, it is deactivated, rendered incapable of activating more clotting factors unless it is reactivated by the enzyme "Vitamin K Epoxide Reductase Complex 1" (VKORC1). Warfarin inhibits VKORC1, thus preventing activation of vitamin K-dependent clotting factors. In simpler terms, warfarin reduces blood clotting by keeping vitamin K in its deactivated form. Since vitamin K is deactivated, it cannot activate certain clotting factors.

Why Antibiotics Interact with Warfarin

Vitamin K enters the body from two sources: the diet (e.g. green leafy vegetables, mayonnaise) and intestinal flora (normal bacteria that reside in the intestine). Intestinal flora produces vitamin K, which gets absorbed into the bloodstream. When antibiotics are introduced into the body, some of the intestinal flora is killed. Since there are fewer bacteria producing vitamin K in the intestine, less vitamin K enters the bloodstream from that source. This results in an exaggerated effect of warfarin, potentially leading to over-anticoagulation and bleeding.

Oral Contraceptives **and** Antibiotics

Antibiotics can decrease the effect of oral contraceptives, which increases the likelihood of contraceptive failure and increases risk of pregnancy. The prevailing theory behind this interaction is reduced enterohepatic circulation of estrogen caused by antibiotic-induced reduction of intestinal flora.

Enterohepatic Circulation of Estrogen

Some estrogen is eliminated by excretion into the bile where is is carried out of the body during defecation. Some of the estrogen that goes into the bile gets hydrolyzed by intestinal flora and subsequently reabsorbed into the blood where it is given another opportunity to exert its pharmacologic effect. Since antibiotics kill intestinal flora, less estrogen gets hydrolyzed and reabsorbed (i.e. the effect of estrogen is reduced).

Vasodilators/Nitrates **and** PDE-5 Inhibitors

Both of these drugs dilate blood vessels. When taken together, blood pressure can drop to a dangerously low level. PDE-5 inhibitors include Viagra® (sildenafil), Levitra® (vardenafil), and Cialis® (tadalafil).

Lithium **and** Diuretics

Lithium is used as a mood stabilizer in psychiatric disorders, and it can also be used to treat/prevent migraine headaches. Lithium is considered to be a "narrow therapeutic index drug," which means that there is less than a 2-fold difference between the median lethal dose and the median effective dose, or there is less than a 2-fold difference between the minimum toxic concentration and the minimum effective concentration. In other words, if the concentration of the drug in the blood gets too high, this therapeutic agent becomes a deadly toxin. The kidneys, which act as a filtration system for the blood, take lithium from the blood so it can leave the body in the urine. Diuretics work by causing the kidneys to transfer more than normal amounts of sodium and water from the blood into the urine. When more sodium is filtered out of the blood by the kidneys, a higher-than-normal amount of lithium is absorbed from the urine back into the blood. As a result, when taking diuretics while on lithium therapy, the concentration of lithium in the blood increases. This can lead to lithium toxicity and, in severe cases, death.

DRUG-FOOD INTERACTIONS

HMG-CoA Reductase Inhibitors (Statins) **and** Grapefruit Juice

Grapefruit juice inhibits the enzyme CYP3A4, a major enzyme involved in the metabolism of certain statins. This elevates the statin levels to higher than normal, leading to increased risk of rhabdomyolysis.

Levodopa **and** Protein

Levodopa is used to treat symptoms of Parkinson's Disease. Dietary protein (e.g. from meat, nuts, and dairy products) interferes with the intestinal absorption of levodopa. Proteins also interfere with levodopa crossing the blood-brain barrier, which levodopa must cross to reach its site of action. As a result, when levodopa is taken with a high protein meal, less levodopa reaches the site of action (the brain).

Warfarin **and** Foods High in Vitamin K*

Since warfarin interferes with the activity of vitamin K, warfarin's effect can be reduced if dietary vitamin K intake increases. As a general rule, patients on warfarin should not avoid vitamin K but should make an effort to be consistent in how much vitamin K they consume each day. *Foods high in vitamin K include: spinach, kale, collard greens, turnip greens, broccoli, Brussels sprouts, mayonnaise, green tea, and canola oil.

Note: Some multivitamins contain vitamin K.

DRUG-DISEASE INTERACTIONS

Decongestants* **and** Hypertension

When sinus blood vessels are swollen and large, they leak fluid and cause sinus congestion. Decongestants provide relief by constricting blood vessels. The blood vessels that are constricted by decongestants are not limited to those located in the sinus passages. Decongestants constrict blood vessels all throughout the body, leading to increased blood pressure. In severe cases, use of a decongestant by an individual with hypertension could result in a cardiovascular event (e.g. stroke, aneurism).

*Decongestants include drugs like Sudafed® (pseudoephedrine) and Sudafed® PE (phenylephrine).

Aspirin **and** Peptic Ulcer Disease

Aspirin has an anti-platelet effect, which predisposes patients to bleeding. This drug is also notorious from causing damage to the lining of the stomach. Patients with peptic ulcer disease have lesions in the lining of their stomach. These lesions can be irritated by aspirin, potentially leading to a gastrointestinal bleed.

DRUG NAME STEMS

When trying to determine the function of a drug, sometimes you will find a clue in the drug name itself. These clues are "drug name stems" and, when present, they usually appear as a suffix in the generic name of a drug. Below are some examples:

-afil = phosphodiesterase 5 (PDE–5) inhibitor (e.g. tadalafil, sildenafil, vardenafil) used to treat erectile dysfunction.

-azepam or **–azolam** = benzodiazepine (e.g. alprazolam, clonazepam, oxazepam, diazepam) used to treat anxiety and/or insomnia.

-azole = antifungal (e.g. clotrimazole, ketoconazole) used to treat fungal infections.

-barbital = barbiturate or barbiturate derivatrive (e.g. phenobarbital, pentobarbital, secobarbital, amobarbital) used to treat seizures.

Ceph- or **Cef-** = cephalosporin antibiotic (e.g. cephalexin, cefazolin, ceftriaxone, ceftazidime, cefdinir) used to treat bacterial infections.

-dronate = bisphosphonate (e.g. ibandronate, alendronate, risedronate) used to treat or prevent osteoporosis.

-floxacin = fluoroquinolone antibiotic (e.g. ciprofloxacin, moxifloxacin, levofloxacin) used to treat bacterial infections.

-gliptin = dipeptidyl peptidase 4 (DPP-4) inhibitor (e.g. saxagliptin, sitagliptin, linagliptin) used to lower blood sugar in type II diabetes mellitus.

-icillin = penicillin antibiotic (e.g. penicillin, amoxicillin, ampicillin, methicillin) used to treat bacterial infections.

-isone = corticosteroid (e.g. prednisone, methylprednisone, hydrocortisone) used to suppress the immune system and reduce inflammation.

-olol = beta-blocker (e.g. metoprolol, atenolol, propranolol, bisoprolol) used to lower blood pressure and/or treat other cardiac conditions such as arrhythmias.

-oprost = prostaglandin analog (e.g. latanoprost) used to treat glaucoma.

-osin = alpha-adrenergic receptor blocker (α-blocker) (e.g. doxazosin, terazosin, prazosin, tamsulosin) used to treat high blood pressure and/or benign prostatic hyperplasia (BPH).

-prazole = proton pump inhibitor (PPI) (e.g. omeprazole, lansoprazole, pantoprazole, rabeprazole) used to suppress stomach acid production.

-pril = angiotensin converting enzyme inhibitor (ACEI) (e.g. lisinopril, benazepril) used to lower blood pressure.

-sartan = angiotensin receptor blocker (ARB) (e.g. valsartan, losartan, olmesartan) used to reduce blood pressure.

-setron = 5-HT_3 (serotonin) antagonist (e.g. ondansetron, palonosetron, granisetron) used to treat or prevent nausea and vomiting (especially nausea and vomiting associated with cancer chemotherapy).

-statin = HMG-CoA reductase inhibitor (e.g. atorvastatin, simvastatin, lovastatin, pravastatin) used to lower cholesterol.

-tidine = H2 receptor blockers (e.g. ranitidine, famotidine, cimetidine) used to suppress stomach acid production.

-triptan = serotonin agonist (5-HT agonist) (e.g. sumatriptan, zolmitriptan, naratriptan, eletriptan) used to treat migraine headaches.

-vir = antiviral (e.g. ritonavir, lopinavir, acyclovir, valacyclovir) used to treat viral infections like shingles, genital herpes, and HIV/AIDS.

NDC NUMBERS

An NDC (National Drug Code) number is an 11-digit number composed of three (3) parts. The first part identifies who manufactured the product, the second part identifies what the product is, and the third part typically identifies the size of the package or the quantity of dosage units contained in the package. The format of an NDC number is as follows:

STRUCTURE OF AN NDC NUMBER

12345–1234–12

FIRST SEGMENT (5 DIGITS)

The first segment of the NDC number identifies the manufacturer of a product (e.g. 00093 is the 5-digit code for TEVA, 52544 represents Watson).

SECOND SEGMENT (4 DIGITS)

The middle segment of the NDC number identifies the product made by the manufacturer (e.g. 0913 is Watson Pharmaceutical's 4-digit code for Norco® 5/325 mg).

THIRD SEGMENT (2 DIGITS)

The last segment of the NDC number usually identifies the package size of the product (e.g. the NDC number for a 100-tablet bottle of Watson's Norco® 5/325 mg is 52544-0913-01 and the NDC number for a 500-tablet bottle is 52544-0913-05).

Note: In most cases, a leading zero is omitted from the NDC number displayed on the label of the manufacturer's stock bottle. For instance, the 11-digit NDC 00093-0287-01 would typically be displayed in one of the following three formats:

0093-0287-01
00093-287-01
00093-0287-1

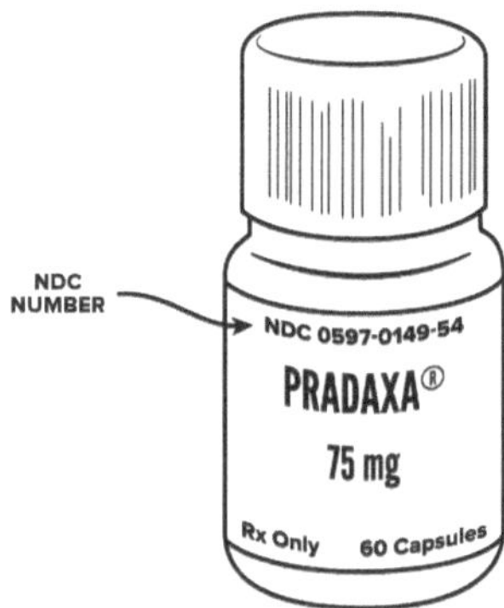

DISPENSING PROCESS

PATIENT PROFILES

Pharmacists need an accurate, up-to-date patient profile for each patient. The information recorded in the patient profile is used for drug interaction screening, patient counseling, and other important functions. The following is a summary of the typical information that pharmacy technicians should record when creating and updating a patient profile:

- Name, address, and phone number
- Date of birth
- Gender
- Prescription Drug Insurance Information
- Health Conditions
- Known allergies
- History of adverse drug reactions
- Complete list of current medications (including OTC drugs & herbal supplements)

As a pharmacy technician, you must make a good faith effort to obtain this information from the patient. If the patient refuses to provide the information, do not argue. Simply document the refusal.

For returning customers, the patient profile should be updated each time the patient drops off a new prescription.

STEP-BY-STEP GUIDE FOR INTERPRETING PRESCRIPTION SIGS

"Sig" is short for the Latin term "signa," which means "to label." On a prescription, the sig is used by the prescriber to communicate the directions for use to the pharmacy. The pharmacy interprets the sig into plain English and places it on the label of the container that will be dispensed to the patient. In most cases, the sig on a prescription (i.e. the directions for use) will be written by the prescriber in abbreviated codes. An example would be: take 1 tab PO BID UD, which is translated by the pharmacy to "take one tablet by mouth twice a day as directed." Many of these abbreviations are derived from Latin or Greek words. For example, BID is an abbreviation for "bis in die," which is Latin for "twice a day." A typical sig is composed of the following parts:

#1 – an action word
(e.g. take, give, instill, apply, place, insert, inject)

#2 – a quantity with units
(e.g. 1 tablet, 2 teaspoonsful, 4 drops, 1 gram, 1 patch, 1 suppository, 5 milliliters)

#3 – a route of administration
(e.g. by mouth, into the left eye, topically to the affected area, to the skin, rectally, vaginally, subcutaneously, intramuscularly, into each nostril, under the tongue)

#4 – the dosing frequency
(e.g. once daily, twice daily, three times daily, four times daily, every 2 hours, every 4 hours, every 6 hours, every 8 hours, every 12 hours, every other day, once a week, once a month)

See the following page for an illustration of a typical prescription.
Pay special attention to the sig.

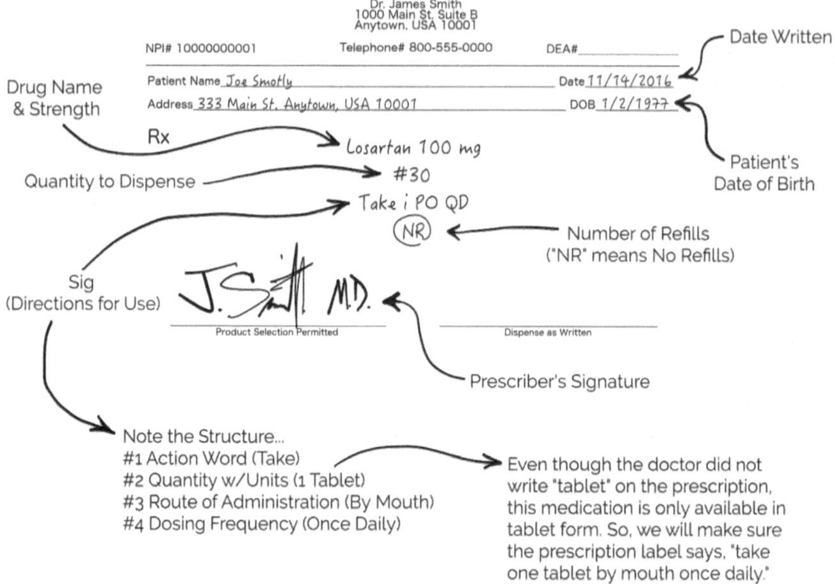

Now that you know what a sig is and what it looks like, memorize the abbreviations and complete the practice problems on the following pages to gain the knowledge and experience needed to translate sig codes competently.

Dosing Frequency

QOD = every other day
QD = every day (daily)
BID = twice daily
TID = three times daily
QID = four times daily
QAM = every morning
QPM = every evening
Qwk = every week
Qmo = every month
H = hours
D = days
SID = once daily (used only by veterinarians)
° = hours (e.g. Q6° = every 6 hours)
hs = bedtime
ac = before meals
cf = with food
wf = with food
pc = after meals
WA = while awake
ATC = around the clock
NTE = not to exceed
PRN = as needed
STAT = immediately

Routes of Administration

PO = by mouth
PR = rectally
PV = vaginally
AU = both ears
AS = left ear
AD = right ear
OU = both eyes
OS = left eye
OD = right eye
IV = intravenous
IVP = intravenous push
IVPB = intravenous piggyback
IM = intramuscular
ID = intradermal
IC = intracardiac
IP = intraperitoneal
IN = intranasal
NG = nasogastric
SQ = subcutaneous
SL = sublingual (under the tongue)
TD = transdermal (across the skin)

Dosing Instructions

UD = as directed
AAA = apply to affected area

Dispensing Instructions

QS = sufficient quantity
NR = no refills
DAW = dispense as written (dispense brand only)

Compounding Instructions

aa = of each
ad = to make; up to
div = divide
qs ad = sufficient quantity to make

Symptoms and Disease States

N/V = nausea and vomiting
HBP = high blood pressure
HTN = hypertension
BPH = benign prostatic hyperplasia (enlarged prostate)
GAD = generalized anxiety disorder
SAD = seasonal affective disorder

Units of Measure
kg = kilogram (one thousand grams)
g = gram
mg = milligram (one one-thousandth of a gram)
μg = microgram (one one-millionth of a gram)
gr = grain (1 grain = 64.8 mg)
gtt = drop
gtts = drops
tsp = teaspoon (5 mL)
tbs = tablespoon (15 mL)
oz = ounce (one fluid ounce = 29.67 mL; one ounce of weight = 28.35 grams)
L = liter
mL = milliliter (one one-thousandth of a liter)
μL = microliter (one one-millionth of a liter)
M = molar
mM = millimolar
mEq = milliequivalent
IU = international unit

Formulations
cr = cream
crm = cream
oint = ointment
ung = ointment
lot = lotion
top = topical
inj = injection
tab = tablet
cap = capsule
susp = suspension
syr = syrup
supp = suppository
CR = controlled release
DR = delayed release
ER = extended release
LA = long acting
SR = sustained release
XR = extended release

Clean Room
PPE = personal protective equipment
D5W = 5% dextrose in water
D10W = 10% dextrose in water
NSS = normal saline solution = 0.9% sodium chloride in water
½ NS = one-half normal saline = 0.45% sodium chloride in water
D5NS = 5% dextrose in normal saline
RL = Ringer's Lactate
LR = Lactated Ringers
SWFI = sterile water for injection
LVP = large volume parenteral (infusion volume greater than 100 mL)
SVP = small volume parenteral (infusion volume equal to or less than 100 mL)
MVI = multivitamin
TPN = total parenteral nutrition

Miscellaneous

USP = United States Pharmacopoeia
NPO = nothing by mouth
D/C = discontinue
c̄ = with
s̄ = without
s̄s̄ = one-half

NKA = no known allergies
NKDA = no known drug allergies
BP = blood pressure
IOP = intraocular pressure
HRT = hormone replacement therapy

Elements/Lab Values

Ca = calcium
Cl = chloride
Fe = iron
K = potassium

Mg = magnesium
Na = sodium
Phos = phosphate
Li = lithium

PRACTICE PROBLEMS

1. Give s̄s̄ tsp PO cf QID x 10D

2. Inj 12 units SQ QHS

3. Insert 1 supp PR Q6H PRN

4. 1 – 2 tabs PO Q4-6H PRN severe pain

5. 1 cap PO up to Q6H PRN N/V

6. AAA on face QPM HS

7. 1 tab PO QD for HTN

8. Inj 0.25 cc IM Qmo UD

9. Instill 1 gtt OS Q2H WA

PRACTICE PROBLEM ANSWERS

1. Give one-half teaspoonful (2.5 mL) by mouth with food 4 times daily for 10 days.
2. Inject 12 units subcutaneously every night at bedtime.
3. Insert one suppository rectally every 6 hours as needed.
4. Take one to two tablets by mouth every 4 to 6 hours as needed for severe pain.
5. Take one capsule by mouth up to every 6 hours as needed for nausea and vomiting.
6. Apply to affected area on face every evening at bedtime.
7. Take one tablet by mouth once daily for hypertension.
8. Inject one-fourth mL (0.25 cc) intramuscularly every month as directed.
9. Instill one drop into left eye every two hours while awake.

COMMON DRUG NAME ABBREVIATIONS

APAP = Acetaminophen
ASA = Aspirin
CPZ = Chlorpromazine
DM = Dextromethorphan
EES = Erythromycin Ethylsuccinate
EPO = Erythropoietin
HC = Hydrocortisone
HCTZ = Hydrochlorothiazide
INH = Isoniazid
KCl = Potassium chloride
MgSO4 = Magnesium sulfate
MMI = Methimazole
MOM = Milk of Magnesia
MSO4 = Morphine sulfate
MTX = Methotrexate
NTG = Nitroglycerin
OC = Oral Contraceptive
PB = Phenobarbital
PCN = Penicillin
PE = Phenylephrine
PSE = Pseudoephedrine
PTU = Propylthiouracil
TAC = Triamcinolone
TCN = Tetracycline

Note: Though commonly used, it is best to avoid abbreviations due to the potential for misinterpretation.

AVOIDING ERRORS

1) Use tall man lettering

Tall man lettering is a way to emphasize the difference in drug names that otherwise look similar. For instance, Hydroxyzine and Hydralazine are two drug names that, at first glance, look quite similar. When you use tall man lettering (HydrOXYzine and HydrALAZINE), the differences in spelling are emphasized, thus reducing the chance that one will be misinterpreted as the other.

Below is a modified list from FDA.gov that demonstrates the use of tall man lettering for look-alike/sound-alike drugs:

AcetaHEXAMIDE	⇔	AcetaZOLAMIDE
BuPROPion	⇔	BusPIRone
ChlorproMAZINE	⇔	ChlorproPAMIDE
ClomiPHENE	⇔	ClomiPRAMINE
CycloSPORINE	⇔	CycloSERINE
DAUNOrubicin	⇔	DOXOrubicin
DimenhyDRINATE	⇔	DiphenhydrAMINE
DOBUTamine	⇔	DOPamine
HydrALAZINE	⇔	HydrOXYzine
MethylPREDNISolone	⇔	MethylTESTOSTERone
NiCARdipine	⇔	NIFEdipine
PredniSONE	⇔	PrednisoLONE
risperiDONE	⇔	rOPINIRole
SulfADIAZINE	⇔	SulfiSOXAZOLE
TOLAZamide	⇔	TOLBUTamide
VinBLAStine	⇔	VinCRIStine

2) Separate inventory

A popular method for preventing medication dispensing errors is separating inventory. When medications are organized alphabetically, it is common to have drugs with very similar names stored right next to each another on the shelf (e.g. Isosorbide Mononitrate & Isosorbide Dinitrate or Metoprolol Tartrate & Metoprolol Succinate). The advantages of separating medications that have similar names are: #1 There is less of a chance that the bottles will get mixed up during storage, and #2 The person filling the prescription is forced to stop and think rather than quickly reach for the first drug that appears to be correct.

3) Use leading zeros

Leading zeros help to ensure accurate translation of numbers less than 1. By omitting a leading zero, you run the risk of causing the patient to receive a dose many times higher than the intended dose. This can be a fatal mistake.

Acceptable: 0.1, 0.005, 0.02, 0.99
Unacceptable: .1, .005, .02, .99

> **What is the difference between .99 and 0.99?**
> .99 could easily be misinterpreted as ninety-nine. Consider how detrimental it would be if a patient was supposed to get 0.99 grams of a drug and they ended up getting 99 grams. One hundred times the prescribed dose. Depending on the drug, an error this big could be fatal.

4) Avoid trailing zeros

While leading zeros can prevent fatal dispensing errors, trailing zeros can cause them. Imagine that a practitioner writes a prescription for Alprazolam 1 mg PO QID PRN anxiety, but when writing the prescription, the practitioner used a trailing zero (one milligram is written as "1.0 mg"). Therefore, the prescription looks like this:

Alprazolam 1.0 mg PO QID PRN anxiety

The decimal point between the number one and the trailing zero is barely visible! When reading this prescription, the technician and pharmacist could easily misinterpret the strength as ten (10) milligrams instead of one (1) milligram. This misinterpretation could lead to a fatal dispensing error. Never use trailing zeros. Write one as 1, not 1.0 or 1.00.

5) Avoid error-prone abbreviations

Another safety strategy is to avoid the use of error-prone abbreviations. Much like leading and trailing zeros, certain abbreviations can lead to dangerous misinterpretations. The FDA and ISMP* have teamed up in a campaign to eliminate the use of error-prone abbreviations. The list below summarizes the most common error-prone abbreviations. Generally, it is best to write out the instructions word for word and avoid abbreviations all together.

ERROR-PRONE ABBREVIATION →	POTENTIAL MISINTERPRETATION
AD (right ear)	OD (right eye)
AS (left ear)	OS (left eye)
AU (both ears)	OU (both eyes)
OD (right eye)	AD (right ear)
OS (left eye)	AS (left ear)
OU (both eyes)	AU (both ears)
CC (cubic centimeters)	U (units)
HS (bedtime)	HS (half-strength) or HR (hour)
BT (bedtime)	BID (twice daily)
IU (international units)	IV (intravenous)
IN (intranasal)	IM (intramuscular)
QD or Q1D (daily)	QID (four times daily)
QOD (every other day)	QD (daily) or QID (four times daily)
OD (right eye)	QD (daily)
SC or SQ (subcutaneous)	5 Q ___ (five every...)
ss (one-half)	55 (fifty-five)
1/D (one per day)	TID (three times daily)
° (hours; e.g. 6° = 6 hours)	0 (zero; e.g. 60 = sixty)
UD (as directed)	Unit Dose
Per Os (by mouth)	OS (left eye)

***What is the ISMP?**

The Institute for Safe Medication Practices (ISMP) is a nonprofit organization devoted to preventing medication errors and ensuring safe use of medications.

6) Read back verbal prescriptions

In certain states (assuming company policy permits), certified pharmacy technicians can accept verbal prescriptions for non-controlled substances from a prescriber (or an agent of the prescriber) over the phone. If you have this privilege/responsibility, always remember to convert the verbal order to writing immediately, write legibly, and read the order back to the prescriber (or the agent of the prescriber) to verify that all of the information was communicated correctly. This is important because, as a good friend of mine says, "What is said is not always the same as what is heard."

7) Promote patient counseling

Patient counseling is the final opportunity to catch a dispensing error before it ends up in the hands of the patient and causes harm. During a patient counseling session, the pharmacist will go over information like the brand and generic name of the medication, what the drug is used to treat, the dose prescribed, etc. Not only is this an opportunity for the patient to receive some basic education on the medicines they take, but it is also an opportunity to identify errors. For instance, let's say you drop-off a prescription for a blood pressure medication. When you go to pick up the medication, the pharmacist explains that the medication is used to treat bacterial infections and then asks you if you have an infection. You say, "No, I have high blood pressure." Disaster averted – the pharmacist realizes that this is a potential dispensing error and takes this opportunity to correct the error before it harms the patient. Even if the patient refuses counseling, at least go over the medication name(s) with them <u>before</u> they purchase the prescription(s).

DAW CODES

Dispense as written (DAW) codes are submitted as part of a third party claim (i.e. the DAW code is communicated to the insurance company during the electronic billing process). The purpose of the DAW code is to describe the reason that the pharmacist selected the brand name product instead of a generic equivalent, or the generic equivalent instead of the brand name product.

DAW 0 = generic substitution permitted by prescriber
DAW 1 = generic substitution not allowed by prescriber
DAW 2 = generic substitution permitted, but patient requested brand product
DAW 3 = generic substitution permitted, but pharmacist selected brand
DAW 4 = generic substitution permitted, but generic not in-stock
DAW 5 = generic substitution permitted, but brand dispensed as generic
DAW 6 = all-purpose override
DAW 7 = law mandated that the brand product be dispensed
DAW 8 = generic substitution permitted, but generic not available on the market
DAW 9 = other

Use the prescription below to answer the questions on the next page.

James Smith, D.O.
Simplified Medical Clinic
10001 N. Main St. Suite 100A, Simple City, USA 24680
Telephone# 123-555-1234

Name John Doe Age 25
Address 111 North Main St. Anywhere, USA 10001 Date 2/27/16

Rx

Bactrim DS
Disp. 20 tablets
Take i PO BID x 10 (ten) days

NR (circled) | 1 | 2 | 3 | 4 | 5 | PRN

James Smith, D.O.

Prescriber must write "Brand Medically Necessary" on the prescription to prohibit generic substitution.

You are billing John Doe's insurance for the Bactrim® DS prescription on the previous page. Since the doctor did not write "Brand Name Medically Necessary" on the prescription, you are going to dispense a generic equivalent (sulfamethoxazole 800 mg/ trimethoprim 160 mg). Which DAW code should you enter for this prescription?
DAW 0.

John Doe leaves the pharmacy to go grocery shopping while his prescription is being filled. When he returns to the pharmacy to pick up his prescription, he insists on getting the brand name version of the medication. Which DAW code would you submit to the insurance in this scenario?
DAW 2.

After Mr. Doe discovers that his insurance will not cover the brand name version of the medication, he tells you that he will go ahead and get the generic version after all. Which DAW code would you submit to the insurance now?
DAW 0.

Which DAW code would you enter if the doctor had written "Brand Name Medically Necessary" on the face of the prescription?
DAW 1.

POP QUIZ

What is Bactrim DS used to treat?
Bacterial infections.

What does the "DS" in Bactrim® DS stand for?
"DS" is an abbreviation for "double strength." Bactrim® is a combination drug, meaning that a single tablet contains two medications. In this case, the two medications are the antibiotics sulfamethoxazole and trimethoprim (sometimes abbreviated as SMZ/TMP or SMX/TMP). One dose of regular strength Bactrim® contains 400 mg of sulfamethoxazole and 80 mg of trimethoprim. One dose of Bactrim® DS contains twice the amount of each active ingredient (800 mg of sulfamethoxazole and 160 mg of trimethoprim). Bactrim® and Bactrim® DS are also available under the brand names Septra® and Septra® DS.

LABELING PRESCRIPTIONS PROPERLY

State* and federal law typically require the following information to appear on the label of a dispensed prescription container:

- Pharmacy's Name, Address & Phone Number
- Rx Number (Prescription Serial Number Generated by the Pharmacy)
- Date the Prescription Was Written, Filled, or Refilled
- Prescriber's Name
- Patient's Name & Address
- Directions for Use
- Precautions, If Written on the Prescription
- Pharmacist's Name or Initials
- Drug Name and Strength
- Drug Manufacturer's (or Distributor's) Name
- Medication Expiration Date (or Beyond-Use Date)

*The requirements vary slightly from state to state.

Note: When labeling a prescription container, ensure all information is visible and legible.

AUXILIARY LABELS

In many cases, the prescriber's directions fall short of providing all of the details necessary for proper use and storage of the prescribed medication. This is where auxiliary labels come in. By affixing the relevant auxiliary labels, pharmacists and pharmacy technicians can help fill in the information gap often left by the prescriber's directions. The computers in most pharmacies are programmed to print the relevant auxiliary labels with each prescription label. See the illustration below for a prescription label with three auxiliary labels (located on the right side of the barcode).

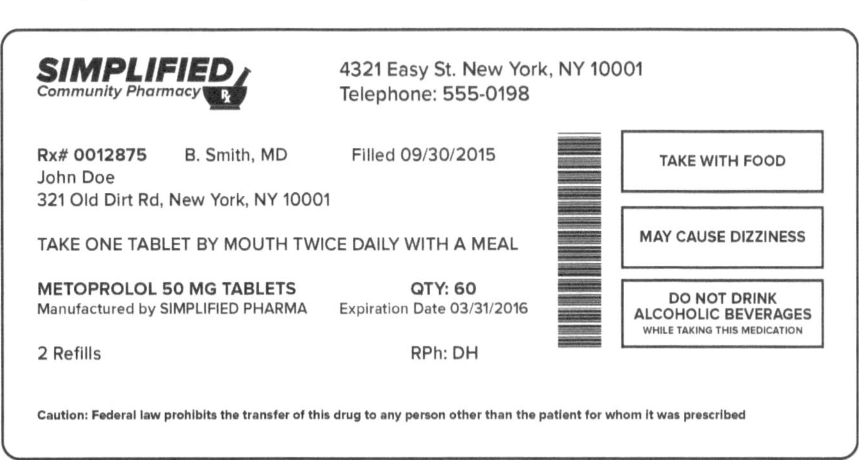

STORAGE REQUIREMENTS

Most medications have specific storage requirements or manufacturer-recommended storage conditions that must be met to ensure the product remains stable and effective until the expiration date. Many environmental factors can negatively affect the chemical structure of the active ingredient(s) and/or disrupt the physical properties of the medium used to deliver the drug into the body (e.g. the drug delivery device and/or the inactive ingredients used to formulate the drug product). The most common examples of these deleterious environmental factors include temperature, humidity/ moisture, and sunlight.

- Temperature
    - Temperature can destroy the chemical and physical properties of a drug product. Study the chart below to learn how terms used in a manufacturer's product packaging like "keep cool" or "store at room temperature" can be translated into quantitative temperature ranges.
- Humidity/Moisture
    - Humidity and moisture can also destroy the chemical and physical properties of a drug product. Study the chart below to learn how terms used in product packaging like "store in a dry place" or "protect from moisture" can be translated into quantitative values.
- Sunlight
    - Sunlight is rich in ultraviolet (UV) light, which has the capacity to change the chemical structure of the active and inactive ingredients that form the drug product. This is why pharmacies use amber vials/containers to dispense medication.

Temperature Ranges	
"Frozen" (Freezer)	-25°C to -10°C (-13°F to 14°F)
"Cold" (Refrigerator)	2°C to 8°C (36°F to 46°F)
"Cool"	8°C to 15°C (46°F to 59°F)
"Room Temperature"	20°C to 25°C (68°F to 77°F)
"Warm"	30°C to 40°C (86°F to 104°F)
"Excessive Heat"	> 40°C (> 104°F)

Humidity Ranges	
"Store in a Dry Place"	Average Relative Humidity < or = 40%
"Protect from Moisture"	Relative Humidity < or = 60%*

*Defined by the World Health Organization (WHO) Technical Report Series.

Drug Products with Special Storage Requirements – Select Examples:

Drug Product	Special Storage Requirement
Nitrostat® (nitroglycerin sublingual tablets)	Do not remove tablets from original container. Nitroglycerin is a volatile substance that quickly converts from solid to gas. When stored outside of the original container, the nitroglycerin will evaporate from the tablet. For this reason, it is important to keep nitroglycerin tablets tightly sealed in the original container (usually a small glass vial with metal lid).
Pradaxa® (dabigatran oral capsules)	Pradaxa® is available in a bottle or blister packs. For the bottle, it is important not to remove the capsules from from their original container until immediately prior to use. The drug is quickly destroyed by humidity in the air. The Pradaxa® bottle is equipped with a special cap that contains a desiccant (drying agent). Once the bottle is opened, the capsules inside expire after 4 months. For the blister packs, do not remove a capsule from the blister pack until immediately prior to use.
Xalatan® (latanoprost eye drops)	Refrigerate (2° – 8°C) until opened. Once opened, latanoprost eye drops can be stored at room temperature (up to 25°C) for 6 weeks.
Insulin (all types and brands)	Refrigerate (2° – 8°C) until first use. Once the rubber stopper of the vial is punctured, it can be stored either in the refrigerator or at room temperature for up to 28 days. After 28 days, sterility cannot be guaranteed.
Nitropress® (sodium nitroprusside injection)	Sodium nitroprusside is quickly deactivated upon exposure to light. To prevent light exposure, the medication comes in a small cardboard box containing a dark amber glass vial of sodium nitroprusside 50 mg/2 mL solution and an opaque light protective sleeve. The vial should only be removed from the box just prior to admixture. Once admixed, the IV infusion bag containing sodium nitroprusside must be placed in the opaque light protective sleeve to prevent exposure to light.

Consequences of Inappropriate Storage – Select Examples:

Product	Consequence
Aerosols *Inhalers* - ProAir®, Ventolin®, Xopenex®, Qvar®, Symbicort® *Rectal Aerosols* - ProctoFoam®, ProctoFoam®-HC *Topical Aerosols* - Kenalog® spray, Tinactin® powder spray	Excessive heat can cause an aerosol container to burst/explode. When used at cool or colder temperatures, aerosol canisters tend to deliver less medication, resulting in suboptimal drug delivery.
Insulin Levemir®, Lantus®, Humulin N®, Novolin N®, Humulin R®, Novolin R®, Humalog®, NovoLog®, Apidra® (and all other forms of insulin)	Insulin is a protein, which is a large molecule whose effectiveness is dependent upon its complex chemical structure. Proteins, such as insulin, have a rather delicate chemical structure. Temperature extremes (heat and cold) and physical shaking can destroy the chemical structure of proteins, rendering them inactive. Additionally, insulin is delivered in a sterile liquid medium as an injection. Warmth and excessive heat promote microbial contamination of the liquid medium, rendering the preparation unsafe for injection.
Suppositories Anucort-HC™ suppositories, Canasa® suppositories, Phenadoz™ suppositories, Glycerin suppositories	A suppository should be maintained in its individual wrapping until directly prior to insertion to protect the dosage form from humidity and moisture in the surrounding environment. If stored outside of their packaging, the suppositories can adhere to one another. Heat and moisture can cause the suppositories to melt and lose form.
Ointments Bactroban® Ointment, Mycolog®-II Ointment, Cortizone-10® Ointment	Warm environments and excessive heat can cause product separation.

Note: The bathroom is one of the worst places to store medication. Why? Hot baths and/or showers create steam (moisture and heat can destroy the ingredient(s)).

PRESCRIPTION DRUG INSURANCE

To submit a claim to a prescription drug insurance plan, you must obtain the following four numbers from the patient's insurance card:

- BIN
- PCN
- Group Number
- ID Number

BIN

BIN stands for Bank Identification Number. The BIN number is a 6-digit number used for processing pharmacy claims electronically. The BIN number identifies the bank or institution that will accept the claim.

PCN

The Processor Control Number (PCN) supplements the information provided by the BIN number. Together with the BIN number, this information functions much like the routing number on a check. The PCN does not have a standardized format; it can vary in length and may be composed of numbers, letters, or a combination of numbers and letters.

Group Number

Many patients obtain medical and prescription drug insurance plans through their employer. The Group Number identifies the employer group or the type of plan to which the patient's plan belongs.

ID Number

The benefits and terms of coverage vary from one person to another, even for people within the same employer group. The Identification Number (ID Number) identifies the patient's individual policy. Together with the group number, this information functions much like the account number on a check.

What is "self-pay?"

"Self-pay" means the patient or customer pays the full cost of the prescription without the help of any third party payers. Depending on which forms of payment your pharmacy accepts, self-pay customers can pay for their prescription(s) using cash, credit card, personal check, etc.

What is a third party payer?

The term "third party payer" refers to an entity outside of the patient-pharmacist relationship that is involved in the financial transaction. The pharmacy is the first party in the transaction, the patient or customer is the second party, and the insurance company (or other payer) is the third party.

What is an insurance claim?

An insurance claim is a request submitted to an insurance company for the payment of a product or service. If the terms of the policy specify coverage of the product or service, then the insurance company will send payment to the provider on behalf of the patient.

What is an insurance premium?
An insurance premium is the cost of maintaining active insurance coverage. When an individual obtains insurance through an employer, the employer deducts the premium from the individual's paycheck. Individuals that obtain insurance on their own also pay their premiums on a periodic basis (e.g. monthly).

What is a deductible?
A deductible is the amount of money a patient must pay out-of-pocket (in addition to the premium) before the insurance benefits are realized. For instance, if "Insurance Plan A" offers 80% co-insurance after a $3,000 annual deductible with a premium of $200/month, then the patient must record $3,000 worth of out-of-pocket medical expenses (in addition to the $200/month premium) before the 80% co-insurance takes effect. In other words, the patient pays 100% of the medical expenses until costs reach $3,000, after which the insurance will pay 80% of medical expenses. This cycle restarts at the beginning of each year.

Note: Typically, insurance policies with a higher deductible have a lower premium and vice versa. For example, an insurance company might offer one policy with a $3,000 annual deductible and a $200/month premium and another policy with a $1,500 annual deductible and a $300/month premium. People who do not believe they will need to use their insurance can increase their deductible, thus lowering their premium. If, in fact, they do not need to use their insurance that year, then they will end up saving money. Of course, no one can predict how much money they will need to spend on medical products and services in a given year.

What is a co-payment?
A co-payment (or "co-pay") is an amount of money paid by the insured individual according to the terms of the insurance policy. For instance, a prescription drug insurance policy might require the patient to pay a $45 co-pay for brand name prescription drugs and a $10 co-pay for generic prescription drugs. The insurance company pays the remaining expense.

What is an HMO?
An HMO (Health Maintenance Organization) is a type of managed care insurance plan. Managed care plans work by forming agreements with healthcare providers. In the agreement, providers adhere to certain treatment guidelines and agree to reimbursement rates set by the HMO. When an HMO insurance plan covers a provider's services, the patients with those plans are more likely to use that provider's services. So, the prescriber benefits by getting to see more patients.

What is a PPO?
A PPO (Preferred Provider Organization) is another type of managed care insurance plan. Like an HMO, a PPO covers medical expenses incurred from healthcare providers and hospitals that have entered into a contract with the PPO. As with an HMO, the provider agrees to certain treatment guidelines and reimbursement rates. Patients with PPO coverage are more likely to visit a covered provider, so the provider benefits from the agreement by getting to see more patients.

What is an insurance formulary?

An insurance formulary is a list of drugs covered under an insurance plan. Insurance companies categorize the covered medications into "tiers." For instance, "tier 1" medications are relatively cheap, highly effective options and are associated with lower co-pays. "Tier 2" medications are usually more expensive options that may have less evidence of benefit and the insurance company charges a higher co-pay for these medications. With each increase in the tier number, the cost of the medication goes up. Generally, the higher the tier, the higher the co-pay.

What is a hospital formulary?

Do not confuse an insurance formulary with a hospital formulary. These are two different things. Instead of managing an overly large inventory of medications, hospitals use a preferred drug list, or "hospital formulary," to determine which medications will be maintained on-hand. For instance, there are several ACE inhibitors on the market, but they all have the same mechanism of action. Rather than try to maintain an inventory that includes every ACE inhibitor, a hospital pharmacy may limit their stock to Lisinopril and Ramipril. When a patient on a different ACE inhibitor (e.g. quinapril) stays at the hospital, they receive one of the ACE inhibitor options from the formulary (Lisinopril or Ramipril). A formulary team composed of physicians, pharmacists, nurses, and other healthcare professionals determines which medications appear on the hospital formulary.

What is CMS?

CMS (Centers for Medicare & Medicaid Services) is the division of the United States Department of Health & Human Services (DHHS) responsible for the administration of government health insurance programs such as Medicare, Medicaid, and SCHIP (State Children's Health Insurance Program).

What is Medicare?

Medicare is a federally funded health insurance program that covers the elderly (age 65 years and older) and people under age 65 with certain disabilities and certain types of kidney disease. There are four (4) parts of Medicare: Part A, B, C, and D.

Medicare Part A

Part A is hospitalization insurance.

Medicare Part B

Medicare Part B covers outpatient medical services, durable medical equipment (e.g. wheelchairs), preventive services (e.g. immunizations), supplies needed to diagnose and treat medical conditions (e.g. blood glucose test strips and lancets for patients with diabetes), and certain medications that are not typically self-administered (e.g. oral cancer chemotherapy drugs and immunosuppressants).

Medicare Part C

Medicare Part C is optional and allows patients to obtain Part A & B coverage through a private insurance company rather than through the federal government. Part C plans are synonymous with "Medicare Advantage Plans."

Medicare Part D
Medicare Part D plans provide optional prescription drug coverage. Private insurance companies administer Medicare Part D plans.

What is Medicaid?
Medicaid is a health insurance and prescription drug insurance plan designed for people of any age with low-income and insufficient resources. Federal and state governments fund Medicaid with tax dollars.

Note: Some patients qualify for both Medicare and Medicaid. Medicaid is the payer of last resort. Bill Medicare as the primary insurance, and Medicaid as the secondary when processing prescriptions for these patients.

What is a prior authorization?
When an insurance company requires "prior authorization," they are essentially refusing to pay a claim until they receive more information from the prescriber. Usually prior authorizations are required when the prescribed drug is expensive and cheaper alternatives exist. When an insurance company requires prior authorization, the pharmacy's role is simply to notify the prescriber, usually by sending a fax. It is the prescriber's responsibility to obtain prior authorization – the pharmacy cannot do this. After the prescriber takes action, the insurance company typically requires an additional 2 – 3 days to process the prior authorization. Even after this process is completed, there is no guarantee the insurance company will pay the claim. Therefore, it is wise to inform the patient that the entire process may take several days, and there is no guarantee that the insurance company will pay the claim. Have the patient contact their insurance company if they have questions, comments, or grievances regarding the prior authorization process.

What is a plan limitation?
Some insurance plans limit the quantity of a medication they will cover. For instance, a plan may only cover a maximum of 15 tablets of zolpidem in a 30-day time period. In these cases, if you try to bill the plan for 16 tablets or more as a 30-days' supply, the claim will be rejected.

What is a Pharmacy Benefits Manager (PBM)?
A Pharmacy Benefits Manager (PBM) is the administrator of the prescription drug portion of a health insurance plan. PBMs enter into contracts* with pharmacies, develop formularies, and process prescription drug claims.

*Pharmacies can only accept insurance payments from insurance companies with which they are contracted. Patients that have insurance from a company not contracted with your pharmacy will not be able to use their insurance at your pharmacy.

What is a Medication Assistance Program (MAP)?
A Medication Assistance Program (MAP) is a program that provides financial help for patients that cannot afford their medications.

How do prescription drug coupons work?

Processing a prescription drug coupon is just like processing insurance claims. The same four numbers are needed (BIN, PCN, group number, and ID number). Many patients present their drug coupons after the filling process is complete. This can disrupt workflow since we have to retrieve the prescription from the pick-up area and reprocess it through the third party payer. To avoid disrupting workflow, ask the patient for any coupons at the drop-off area.

Note: Patients enrolled in government prescription drug insurance programs, such as Medicaid or Medicare Part D, cannot use prescription drug coupons. In addition, each coupon has its own fine print (terms & conditions) that may restrict use.

What is "coordination of benefits?"

Coordination of benefits is necessary when billing two or more third party payers at the same time. In these cases, we must take measures to ensure each payer pays the proper amount – we cannot charge each payer for the full amount of the claim. Coordinating the benefits means charging the full amount to the primary payer and only the remainder to the secondary payer, and so on. Intentionally or unintentionally obtaining overpayment or duplicate payments is a form of insurance fraud.

SUMMARY OF COMMON INSURANCE (THIRD PARTY) CLAIM REJECTIONS AND POTENTIAL SOLUTIONS:

- **Rejection Reason:** Non-Formulary Medication
    - **Solution:** The medication is not covered by the patient's plan. Fax the prescriber to request a substitute or ask the patient if they would like to self-pay.
- **Rejection Reason:** NDC Not Covered
    - **Solution:** Try filling the prescription using a different manufacturer.
- **Rejection Reason:** Refill Too Soon
    - **Solution:** Find the next refill date in the rejection details. Notify the patient and re-submit the claim on the next refill date.
- **Rejection Reason:** Invalid Days' Supply
    - **Solution:** Search the rejection details for days' supply limits. If appropriate, change the dispensed quantity so that the days' supply falls within the limits enforced by the insurance plan. Notify the patient of any changes.
- **Rejection Reason:** Prior Authorization Required
    - **Solution:** Fax the prescriber to notify him/her that prior authorization is required. Include the prescription information and the insurance company's phone number.
- **Rejection Reason:** Therapeutic duplication*
- **Rejection Reason:** Drug-drug interaction*
- **Rejection Reason:** Drug utilization review (DUR)*
- **Rejection Reason:** Look-alike/sound-alike*
- **Rejection Reason:** Dose too high*

*These rejections must be addressed by a pharmacist.

MEASUREMENT SYSTEMS

There are three (3) systems of measurement used in pharmacy.

1. The apothecaries' system
2. The avoirdupois system
3. The metric system

The Apothecaries' System

Used in ancient Greece, the apothecaries' system is for the most part outdated, but a few older drugs do still have their strengths expressed in units of grains. Examples include: aspirin, ferrous sulfate, Armour Thyroid, nitroglycerin, and phenobarbital. In this system, the grain is the smallest unit of weight, and the minim is the smallest unit of volume.

Weight
1 grain (gr) = 64.8 milligrams
1 scruple (℈) = 20 grains
1 dram (ʒ) = 3 scruples
1 ounce (℥) = 8 drams
1 pound = 12 ounces

Volume
1 minim (♏) ~ 0.0617 mL
1 fluid dram = 60 minims
1 fluid ounce = 8 fluid drams
1 pint = 16 fluid ounces
1 quart = 2 pints
1 gallon = 4 quarts

The Avoirdupois System

The avoirdupois measurement system is the customary system of weights and measures in the United States. In this system, one (1) pound equals 16 ounces.

Weight
1 grain = 64.8 mg
1 ounce (oz) = 437.5 grains
1 pound lb) = 16 ounces

Volume
1 fluid ounce = 29.57 mL
1 cup = 8 fluid ounces
1 pint = 2 cups
1 quart = 2 pints
1 gallon = 4 quarts

The Metric System

The metric system is the standard measurement system for pharmacy and medicine. As a base ten system, it is also the simplest measurement system.

Weight
1 milligram (mg) = 1,000 micrograms
1 gram (g) = 1,000 milligrams
1 kilogram (kg) = 1,000 grams

Volume
1 milliliter (mL) = 1 cm^3 (cc)
1 deciliter (dL) = 100 milliliters
1 liter (L) = 1,000 milliliters

ROMAN NUMERALS

ROMAN NUMERALS
I = 1
V = 5
X = 10
L = 50
C = 100
D = 500
M = 1,000

Rules

1) When Roman numerals are repeated, add them together.
    - Example: III = I + I + I = 3
2) When a smaller Roman numeral is written to the right of a larger Roman numeral, add them together.
    - Example: VI = V + I = 6
3) When a smaller Roman numeral is written to the left of a larger Roman numeral, subtract it from the larger Roman numeral.
    - Example IX = X – I = 9
4) Do not use more than three of the same Roman numeral in a sequence.
    - Example: ~~IIII = 4~~ IV = 4
5) When rule 2 and 3 are in conflict, use rule 3.
    - Example: ~~XIX = 21~~ XIX = 19

Examples

Roman numeral XII = 12
Roman numeral XXIV = 24
Roman numeral LIX = 59

PRACTICE PROBLEMS

Convert these numbers to Roman numerals:

1. 120
2. 80
3. 30
4. 3750
5. 1200
6. 473
7. 15
8. 291

Convert these Roman numerals to numbers:

9. CL
10. XC
11. LXV
12. XLVIII
13. MM
14. CCXL
15. CDLXXX
16. CCLVI

PRACTICE PROBLEM ANSWERS

1. CXX
2. LXXX
3. XXX
4. MMMDCCL
5. MCC
6. CDLXXIII
7. XV
8. CCXCI
9. 150
10. 90
11. 65
12. 48
13. 2000
14. 240
15. 480
16. 256

AVERAGES

There are three ways to express an average: Mean, Median, and Mode.

Mean – Add up all the values and divide by the number of values.

Example

Seven values are given: 1, 4, 6, 3, 9, 8, 3

Add the seven values: 1 + 4 + 6 + 3 + 9 + 8 + 3 = 34

Divide by seven: 34 ÷ 7 = 4.9

Mean = 4.9

Median – Identify the middle value.

Example

Nine values are given: 11, 3, 10, 5, 4, 5, 5, 8, 7

Rearrange values into chronological order: 3, 4, 5, 5, 5, 7, 8, 10, 11

Determine the middle number: 3, 4, 5, 5, **5**, 7, 8, 10, 11

Median = 5

Mode – Identify the value that appears most often in a set of values.

Example

Eight values are given: 4, 6, 7, 1, 3, 1, 3, 1

Tally the number of times each value is presented and identify the most commonly presented value:

1: III

3: II

4: I

6: I

7: I

Mode = 1

EXAMPLE PROBLEM

A patient measured her blood glucose level daily for one week. Based on her measurements, what was her mean blood glucose for the week?

Monday: 190 mg/dL

Tuesday: 182 mg/dL

Wednesday: 110 mg/dL

Thursday: 90 mg/dL

Friday: 125 mg/dL

Saturday: 130 mg/dL

Sunday: 70 mg/dL

Solution:

$$\frac{(190 + 182 + 110 + 90 + 125 + 130 + 70)\ \text{mg/dL}}{7} = 128\ \text{mg/dL}$$

Answer: 128 mg/dL

PRACTICE PROBLEMS

1. What is the median in the following set of numbers: 19, 12, 49, 34, 101, 67, 1?

2. What is the mode in the following set of numbers: 4, 2, 1, 4, 5, 2, 4, 3, 2, 1, 2, 4, 2?

3. What is the mean in the following set of numbers: 3, 1, 4, 5, 2, 3, 5, 1, 5, 3, 2, 2, 4?

PRACTICE PROBLEM ANSWERS

1. 34
2. 2
3. 3.1

DENSITY AND SPECIFIC GRAVITY

Density = mass (grams) per unit volume (milliliters).

$$\text{Density} = \frac{\text{Mass (grams)}}{\text{Volume (milliliters)}}$$

Specific gravity = the density of a substance relative to the density of a reference substance*.

$$\text{Specific Gravity} = \frac{\text{Density of Substance}}{\text{Density of Reference Substance}}$$

*The reference substance is usually H_2O (water), which has a density of 1 g/mL. When water is the reference substance, the specific gravity is the same value as the density but without units. For example, the density of glycerin is 1.26 g/mL. When you calculate the specific gravity of glycerin, you take the density of glycerin and divide that by the density of water (1.26 g/mL ÷ 1 g/mL = 1.26). Essentially all that happens is the units cancel out. The specific gravity of glycerin = 1.26.

EXAMPLE PROBLEMS

You weigh 30 mL of a mystery substance to determine its identity. If the 30 mL sample of the substance weighs 33.3 grams, what is the identity of the substance?

A. Water (Density = 1. 0 g/mL)
B. Isopropyl Alcohol (Density = 0.79 g/mL)
C. Glycerin (Density = 1.26 g/mL)
D. Simple Syrup (Density = 1.3 g/mL)
E. Ethylene Glycol (Density = 1.11 g/mL)

Solution:

$$\text{Density} = \frac{\text{Mass (g)}}{\text{Volume (mL)}} = \frac{33.3\text{ g}}{30\text{ mL}} = 1.11\text{ g/mL}$$

Answer: E. Ethylene Glycol (Density = 1.11 g/mL)

To compound 60 grams of a formulation that contains 10% (w/w) petrolatum, how many milliliters of pure melted liquid petrolatum would be required?
Note: Density of petrolatum = 0.9 g/mL

Solution:

$$\frac{10 \text{ parts of petrolatum}}{100 \text{ parts total}} \text{ x } 60 \text{ g total formulation} = 6 \text{ g of petrolatum}$$

$$6 \text{ g of petrolatum x } \frac{\text{mL}}{0.9 \text{ g}} = 6.67 \text{ mL of petrolatum}$$

Answer: 6.67 mL of petrolatum

PRACTICE PROBLEMS

1. How much does 4 mL of a substance weigh if its density is 1.2 g/mL?

2. What volume of simple syrup (density 1.3 g/mL) would be needed to obtain a sample that weighs 2 grams?

3. What would the specific gravity of water be (density = 1 g/mL) if the reference substance was glycerin (density = 1.26 g/mL)?

4. If 78 mL of Substance H weighs 131 grams, what is the density of Substance H?

5. If 12 grams of Liquid Q occupies a volume of 15 mL, what is the specific gravity of Liquid Q (assume reference substance is water)?

PRACTICE PROBLEM ANSWERS

1. 4.8 g
2. 1.54 mL
3. 0.79
4. 1.68 g/mL
5. 0.8

TEMPERATURE CONVERSION

A temperature conversion problem will be easy points on the ExCPT exam... if you know how to solve it. Memorize the equations for converting Fahrenheit to Celsius and Celsius to Fahrenheit and know how to apply them.

CONVERTING FROM FAHRENHEIT TO CELSIUS:

$$°C = \frac{5}{9}\ (°F - 32)$$

CONVERTING FROM CELSIUS TO FAHRENHEIT:

$$°F = \left(\frac{9}{5} \times °C\right) + 32$$

TEMPERATURE CONVERSION VALUES TO MEMORIZE

Freezing Point of Water: 0°C = 32°F
Human Body Temperature: 37°C = 98.6°F
Boiling Point of Water: 100°C = 212°F

EXAMPLE PROBLEM

You read that insulin should be stored at 2 – 8°C. What is this temperature range in degrees Fahrenheit?

Solution:

$$\left(\frac{9}{5} \times 2°C\right) + 32 = 36°F \qquad \left(\frac{9}{5} \times 8°C\right) + 32 = 46°F$$

Answer: 36 – 46°F

PRACTICE PROBLEMS

Convert to Fahrenheit:

1) –3°C
2) 0°C
3) 1°C
4) 6°C
5) 25°C
6) 60°C

Convert to Celsius:

7) –10°F
8) 0°F
9) 32°F
10) 98.6°F
11) 72°F
12) 101°F

PRACTICE PROBLEM ANSWERS

1) 27°F
2) 32°F
3) 34°F
4) 43°F
5) 77°F
6) 140°F

7) -23°C
8) -18°C
9) 0°C
10) 37°C
11) 22°C
12) 38.3°C

INTRODUCTION TO PROPORTIONS AND UNIT CONVERSION

Most of the math you will face on the ExCPT exam involves proportions. The following is an example of a proportion:

$$\frac{a}{b} = \frac{c}{d}$$

When you get a proportion problem, you must first cross multiply. For example:

$$\frac{a}{b} = \frac{c}{d} \therefore a \times d = b \times c$$

Then isolate the unknown. For instance:

$$a = \frac{b \times c}{d} \quad \text{or} \quad b = \frac{a \times d}{c} \quad \text{or} \quad c = \frac{a \times d}{b} \quad \text{or} \quad d = \frac{b \times c}{a}$$

Here is an example of a real-life problem that involves proportions:
A car travels at a speed of 60 miles per hour. How many miles does the car travel in 2.5 hours?

$$\frac{60 \text{ miles}}{1 \text{ hour}} = \frac{? \text{ miles}}{2.5 \text{ hours}} \therefore ? \text{ miles} = \frac{60 \text{ miles} \times 2.5 \text{ hours}}{1 \text{ hour}} = 150 \text{ miles}$$

Be sure that the units match on each side of the proportion. For instance, let's say the question was: how many miles were traveled in 150 minutes?

To solve this problem, you would first need to convert the units from minutes to hours like this:

$$150 \text{ minutes} \times \frac{1 \text{ hour}}{60 \text{ minutes}} = 2.5 \text{ hours}$$

These units cancel out.

Many pharmacy calculations are quickly solved using the same approach. For instance, let's say you dispense 50 tablets to a patient that takes 2 tablets per day. How many days will the bottle of 50 tablets last?

$$50 \text{ tablets} \times \frac{\text{day}}{2 \text{ tablets}} = 25 \text{ days}$$

The term 1 hour/60 minutes is a "conversion factor." When we multiplied 150 minutes by 1hour/60 minutes, we essentially multiplied the value 150 minutes by a factor of 1. Why? Because this calculation did not increase or decrease the amount of time the car was traveling; it just changed the units used to express the amount of time traveled (150 minutes and 2.5 hours are the same thing). You will use conversion factors frequently when solving pharmacy math problems. For instance, one conversion factor commonly used in pharmacy is 5 milliliters/teaspoonful (can also be expressed as 1 teaspoonful/5 milliliters). You need to memorize this conversion factor and a few others (see the list of **Must-Know Conversion Factors** in the section titled "The Secret to Solving Nearly Any Pharmacy Math Problem").

THE SECRET TO SOLVING NEARLY ANY PHARMACY MATH PROBLEM

The secret is simple – in fact, we have already begun to reveal the secret – it is simply unit conversion. Many textbooks try to teach a more complex version of this concept that is unnecessarily difficult. The approach I am about to teach you is the same one that I successfully use to solve nearly *all* of the problems I encounter in my everyday work. The best advice to mastering this approach is to work through a lot of examples and practice problems (plenty of which you will find on the following pages). You will see this problem-solving approach applied throughout this study guide. First, ***memorize*** the **Must-Know Conversion Factors** (listed below) and the **Common Pharmacy Math Equations** (listed in *Appendix A* in the back of the book). Then, move on to the next page and begin solving real-world pharmacy problems! Below is the general equation you will use:

(# in Given Units) x (Conversion Factor*) = # in Desired Units

*Conversion Factor = Desired Units/Given Units

MUST-KNOW CONVERSION FACTORS:

VOLUME
1 cubic centimeter (cc) = 1 milliliter (mL)
1 Liter (L) = 1,000 mL
1 teaspoon (tsp) = 5 mL
1 tablespoon (tbsp) = 3 tsp = 15 mL
1 fluid ounce (volume) = 29.57 mL*
**Most pharmacists round up to 30 mL*
1 Cup = 8 fluid ounces (fl oz)
1 Pint = 2 cups
1 Quart = 2 pints
1 Gallon = 4 quarts

WEIGHT
1 milligram (mg) = 1,000 micrograms
1 gram (g) = 1,000 mg
1 kilogram (kg) = 1,000 g
1 kg = 2.2 pounds (lb)
1 ounce (oz) = 28.35 g
1 lb = 454 g
1 grain (gr) = 64.8 mg

HEIGHT
1 inch (in) = 2.54 centimeters (cm)

Solving pharmacy math problems is all about combining what you are given with what you know to get where you need to go.

1) What you are given:
   The information provided in the problem/question.
2) What you know:
   The **Must-Know Conversion Factors** and the **Common Pharmacy Math Equations.**
3) Where you need to go:
   What to do with the information now that you have collected it.

EXAMPLE PROBLEM

A 5 year-old child has a cardiac arrhythmia. To treat the arrhythmia, the doctor prescribes propranolol at the daily dose of 0.5 mg/kg. If we determine that the child weighs 55 pounds, how many milligrams of propranolol should the child receive each day?

What you are given:
Age = 5 years old
Dose = 0.5 mg/kg
Weight = 55 lb

What you know:
Must-Know Conversion Factors
Common Pharmacy Math Equations

Where to go:
Using what you are given and what you know, you must determine how many milligrams of the medication the patient should receive each day. Everything you need to solve the problem will come from what you are given and/or what you know. All you have to do is take this information and make the units change and/or cancel out until you get the desired units.

The dose is already given in the question as 0.5 mg/kg. Now, just find a way to get the kilogram units to cancel out, and then you will have the dose in milligrams.

$$\frac{0.5\text{ mg}}{\text{kg}} \times ? \times ?\ldots = ?\text{ mg}$$

$$\frac{0.5\ mg}{kg} \times ? \times ?... = ?\ mg$$

What factor(s) must you multiply by to get an answer in milligrams?

Now is the time to look back at "what you are given" and "what you know"to pick out the factors you will be able to use to cancel out the kilogram units and obtain your answer in milligrams.

What you are given:
~~Age = 5 years old~~ (age is irrelevant, because the dose is based on weight)

Dose = 0.5 mg/kg

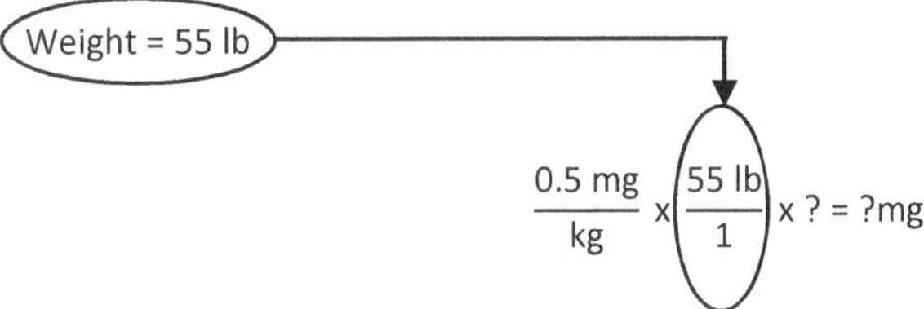

You are given the child's weight in the question. If only the weight was in units of kilograms, then you would be able to solve the problem.

What you know:

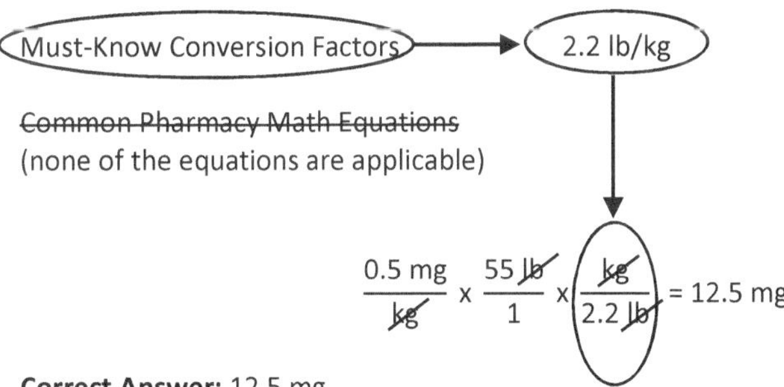

Correct Answer: 12.5 mg

The key to solving this problem was taking what you were given, combining it with what you know, and then figuring out what information/which pieces of information was/were relevant for obtaining the desired units.

MORE EXAMPLE PROBLEMS

How many fluid ounces (℥) are in 118 mL (please answer in Roman numerals)?

Solution:

Think of the dividing line as the word "per"

$$\text{\# in Desired Units} = 118 \text{ mL} \times \frac{1 \text{ fluid ounce}}{29.57 \text{ mL}} = 4 \text{ fluid ounces}$$

Note: notice how the mL units cancel out.

Answer: IV ℥ (4 fluid ounces)

***There are 29.57 milliliters **per** fluid ounce (29.57 mL/fluid ounce). This can be written as "29.57 mL/1 fluid ounce" **or** "1 fluid ounce/29.57 mL." Since 1 fluid ounce is *equal* to 29.57 mL, then 29.57 mL ÷ 1 fluid ounce = 1.

Multiplying a value by the factor "29.57 mL/1 fluid ounce" is like multiplying it by 1. The actual value doesn't change, but the units do change. This is true when you multiply any number by a conversion factor.

Since multiplying by the factor "29.57 mL/1 fluid ounce" is mathematically the same as multiplying by 1, multiplying the reciprocal "1 fluid ounce/29.57 mL" is also like multiplying by 1. How do you know which way to orient the conversion factor? You have to decide which units you want on top (the numerator) and which units you want on the bottom (the denominator) based on what units you are trying to obtain. The units you are trying to obtain should go in the numerator and the units you are trying to eliminate should go in the denominator. See below for an example of what happens when you orient the conversion factor ***the wrong way***:

$$118 \text{ mL} \times \frac{29.57 \text{ mL}}{1 \text{ fluid ounce}} = 3{,}489 \text{ mL}^2/\text{fluid ounce}$$

...clearly, this did not give us the units we were looking for.

How many kilograms (kg) does a 77 lb patient weigh?

Solution:

$$\text{\# in Desired Units} = 77 \text{ lb} \times \frac{\text{kg}}{2.2 \text{ lb}} = 35 \text{ kg}$$

Answer: 35 kg

How many milliliters are in 16 ounces?

Solution:

$$\# \text{ in Desired Units} = 16 \text{ ounces} \times \frac{29.57 \text{ mL}}{\text{ounce}} = 473 \text{ mL}$$

Note: Milliliters (mL) are the "Desired Units" because the question asks for an answer in milliliters. Likewise, the # in Given Units is 16 ounces, as that is the value we are given. Since we know the conversion factor (29.57 mL per ounce), we have all the information needed to solve the problem.

Answer: 473 mL

A patient drops off a prescription for 30 tablets of 5 grain ferrous sulfate. You only have four iron products stocked in the pharmacy. Which of the four products should you dispense?

A. Fergon® (Ferrous gluconate 250 mg)
B. Ferro-Sequels® (Ferrous fumarate 150 mg)
C. Feosol® (Ferrous sulfate 325 mg)
D. SlowFe® (Ferrous sulfate 225 mg)

Solution:

$$\# \text{ in Desired Units} = \frac{5 \text{ grains}}{1} \times \frac{64.8 \text{ mg}}{\text{grain}} = 324 \text{ mg}$$

Answer: C. Feosol® (Ferrous sulfate 325 mg)

Note: The answer we calculated was 1 mg lower than the answer we selected. Why is this alright? Many times, the value of 1 grain is rounded up to 65 mg. If you were to use 1 grain = 65 mg as the conversion factor (rather than 1 grain = 64.8 mg), your answer would be 325 mg. The difference is not significant, so either strength is acceptable.

You receive a prescription order for Nitrostat® sublingual tablets 1/200 grain. Nitrostat® sublingual tablets are available in 3 strengths. Which strength should you dispense?

A. 0.3 mg
B. 0.4 mg
C. 0.6 mg

Solution:

$$\# \text{ in Desired Units} = \frac{1 \text{ grain}}{200} \times \frac{64.8 \text{ mg}}{\text{grain}} = 0.3 \text{ mg}$$

Answer: A. 0.3 mg

An order comes to the pharmacy for levothyroxine 0.125 mg IV injection. Using a levothyroxine 40 mcg/mL solution, how many milliliters should you dispense?

A. 0.0031 mL
B. 3.1 mL
C. 0.31 mL
D. 3.1 µL

Solution:

$$\text{\# in Desired Units} = \frac{0.125 \text{ mg}}{1} \times \frac{1{,}000 \text{ mcg}}{\text{mg}} \times \frac{\text{mL}}{40 \text{ mcg}} = 3.1 \text{ mL}$$

Answer: B. 3.1 mL

A patient weighs 100.1 kg. What is the patient's weight in pounds?

Solution:

$$\text{\# in Desired Units} = \frac{100.1 \text{ kg}}{1} \times \frac{2.2 \text{ lb}}{\text{kg}} = 220 \text{ lb}$$

Answer: 220 lb

The Glucagon Emergency Kit for Low Blood Sugar, manufactured by Lilly, comes with a vial containing 1 mg of glucagon and 49 mg of lactose. Assuming Lilly has all the glucagon it needs, how many vials can they prepare using only one pound of lactose?

$$\frac{1 \text{ lb of lactose}}{1} \times \frac{16 \text{ ounces}}{\text{pound}} \times \frac{28.35 \text{ g}}{\text{ounce}} \times \frac{1{,}000 \text{ mg}}{\text{g}} = 453{,}600 \text{ mg of lactose}$$

$$\frac{453{,}600 \text{ mg of lactose}}{1} \times \frac{\text{vial}}{49 \text{ mg of lactose}} = 9{,}257 \text{ vials}$$

Answer: 9,257 vials

Sometimes the conversion factor is given in the question. For example:

What is the days' supply of a bottle of 90 tablets of levothyroxine 112 mcg if the instructions are to take one tablet by mouth every day, except take one-half tablet on Sundays?

Solution:

$$\frac{90\ \text{tablets}}{1} \times \frac{7\ \text{days}}{6.5\ \text{tablets}} = 96.9\ \text{days} \therefore 97\ \text{days}$$

Note: The conversion factor here was 6.5 tablets/7 days.

Answer: 97 days

Given a solution that contains 100 mg of drug per 5 mL, how many milliliters would be required to obtain a dose of 650 mg?

Solution:

$$\frac{650\ \text{mg}}{1} \times \frac{5\ \text{mL}}{100\ \text{mg}} = 32.5\ \text{mL}$$

Answer: 32.5 mL

Sometimes, you will need to do a series of conversions to reach the answer you need. Take this problem for example: How many 75 mcg tablets can be made from six pounds of a drug?

Solution:

$$\frac{6\ \text{pounds}}{1} \times \frac{16\ \text{ounces}}{\text{lb}} \times \frac{28.35\ \text{g}}{\text{ounce}} \times \frac{1{,}000{,}000\ \text{mcg}}{\text{g}} \times \frac{\text{tablet}}{75\ \text{mcg}} = 36{,}288{,}000\ \text{tablets}$$

Answer: 36,288,000 tablets

PRACTICE PROBLEMS

1. How many fluid ounces are in a jug containing 3,785 mL of polyethylene glycol with electrolytes?

2. After reconstitution, how many teaspoons are in three 100-mL bottles of Amoxicillin 250 mg/5 mL oral suspension? Express your answer in Roman numerals.

3. Approximately how many tablespoons are in a 4 oz bottle of cough syrup?

4. How many scruples of aspirin are in sixteen 5 grain tablets of Ecotrin®?

5. If a patient is 6 feet tall, how tall would the patient be in centimeters?

6. You have 7 pounds of triamcinolone 0.1% ointment. How many kilograms do you have?

7. How many tablespoons are in a 150-mL bottle of an antibiotic suspension?

8. How many milliliters of a 200 mg/mL solution of testosterone cypionate should be injected intramuscularly if the patient needs to receive 75 mg per injection?

9. How many milliliters are needed to provide one 300 mg dose of amoxicillin using a 250 mg/5 mL amoxicillin suspension?

10. If a patient applies 4 g of Voltaren® 1% Gel (10 mg diclofenac/1 g gel) to her knee every day then how many milligrams of diclofenac are being applied daily?

11. A physician wrote a prescription for testosterone cypionate 200 mg/mL solution with the instructions to inject 0.75 mL intramuscularly once every two weeks. How many grams of the drug will the patient inject over the course of one year?

PRACTICE PROBLEM ANSWERS

1. 128 fluid ounces
2. LX teaspoons
3. 8 tablespoons
4. 4 scruples
5. 183 centimeters
6. 3.18 kilograms
7. 10 tablespoons
8. 0.375 milliliters
9. 6 mL
10. 40 mg
11. 3.9 g

MILLIEQUIVALENTS

Most units of measure can be converted simply by multiplying by the appropriate conversion factor, but milliequivalents (mEq) are the exception to the rule. Milligrams are similar to milliequivalents, but with one simple distinction - milligrams are a measure of mass, whereas milliequivalents are a measure of the concentration of ions. To convert between milligrams (mg) and mEq, use the following equations:

CONVERT FROM mg TO mEq

$$\frac{\text{mg} \times \text{Valence}}{\text{Molecular Weight}} = ?\ \text{mEq}$$

CONVERT FROM mEq TO mg

$$\frac{\text{mEq} \times \text{Molecular Weight}}{\text{Valence}} = ?\ \text{mg}$$

Molecular weight is determined by adding the atomic mass of each element in a molecule. You can find atomic mass values in the periodic table. Valence values can be determined from their location in periodic table, but we created the following chart to summarize the molecular weight and valence values for the most common electrolytes seen in pharmacy practice:

Electrolyte	Valence	Molecular Weight
Calcium (Ca^{2+})	2	40
Ferrous (Fe^{2+})	2	56
Ferric (Fe^{3+})	3	56
Lithium (Li^{+})	1	7
Magnesium (Mg^{2+})	2	24
Potassium (K^{+})	1	39
Sodium (Na^{+})	1	23
Carbonate (CO_3^{2-})	2	60
Chloride (Cl^{-})	1	35.5
Sulfate (SO_4^{2-})	2	96

EXAMPLE PROBLEMS

How many milligrams of potassium chloride are in one 20 mEq tablet of potassium chloride (K-Dur®)?

A. 710 mg
B. 780 mg
C. 1,490 mg
D. 1,560 mg

Solution:

$$\frac{\text{mEq} \times \text{Molecular Weight}}{\text{Valence}} = ?\ \text{mg} \qquad \frac{20\ \text{mEq} \times (39 + 35.5)}{1} = 1{,}490\ \text{mg}$$

Answer: C. 1,490 mg

How many milliequivalents are in 3.54 grams of sodium?

A. 1.54 mEq
B. 3.08 mEq
C. 154 mEq
D. 308 mEq

Solution:

$$\frac{\text{mg} \times \text{Valence}}{\text{Molecular Weight}} = ?\ \text{mEq} \qquad \frac{3{,}540\ \text{mg} \times 1}{23} = 154\ \text{mEq}$$

Answer: C. 154 mEq

INTRODUCTION TO COMPOUNDING

What is compounding?

In a way, compounding is like manufacturing on a very small scale; however, legislators have gone to great lengths to make distinctions between compounding and manufacturing. Compounding can take place in a registered pharmacy under the supervision of a licensed pharmacist, but manufacturing cannot. Likewise, manufacturing can take place in a facility that is registered as a drug manufacturing business, but compounding cannot. So, what exactly is compounding then? Compounding is the creation of personalized, *patient-specific* medications. For instance, a patient who is unable to swallow pills may need to receive a drug that is only available commercially as an oral tablet. In cases like this, the pharmacy may be called upon to compound a customized version of the medication (e.g. an oral liquid version of the medication).

How does the law distinguish between compounding pharmacies and manufacturers?

Compounding pharmacies must adhere to these basic guidelines (among others):

- A compounded drug product cannot be a copy of a commercially available FDA-approved product.
- A compounded drug product cannot contain any ingredient that has been deemed unsafe or ineffective.
- Products can only be compounded after receiving an individual, patient-specific prescription order (or in anticipation of receiving a patient-specific prescription order where an established prescribing pattern exists).

Now that you understand what compounding is, let's take a look at some standard compounding equipment and the math you will need to use when compounding a drug product.

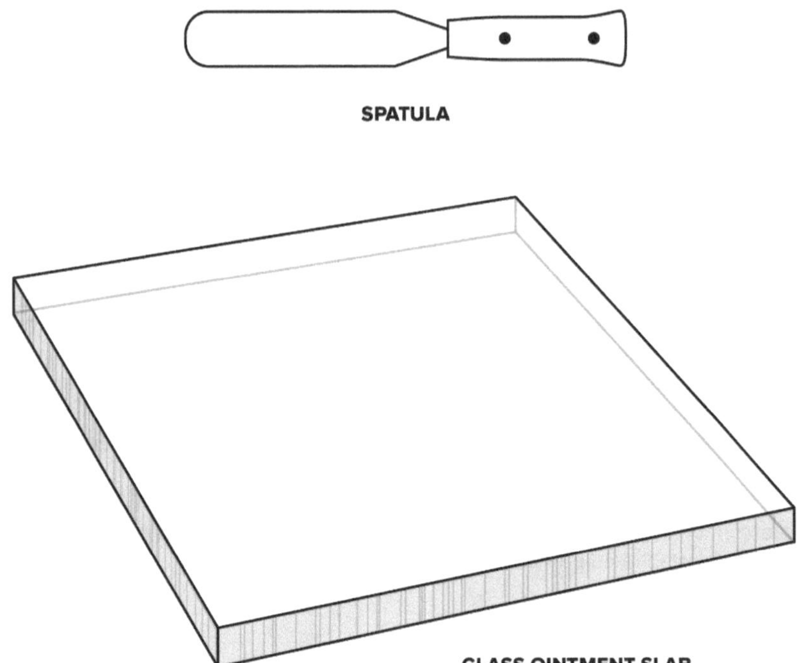
SPATULA
GLASS OINTMENT SLAB

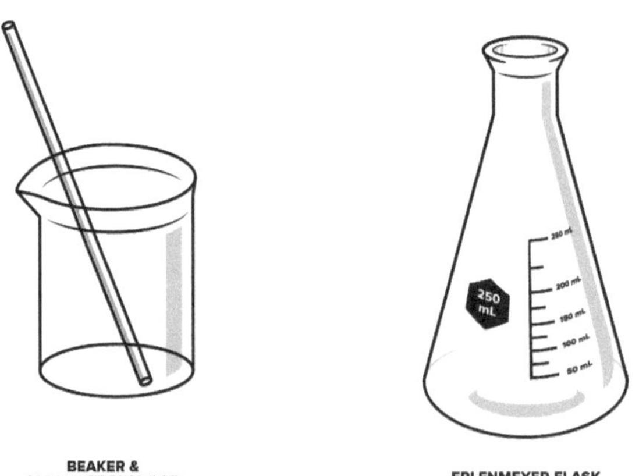
250 mL
BEAKER &
GLASS STIRRING ROD
ERLENMEYER FLASK

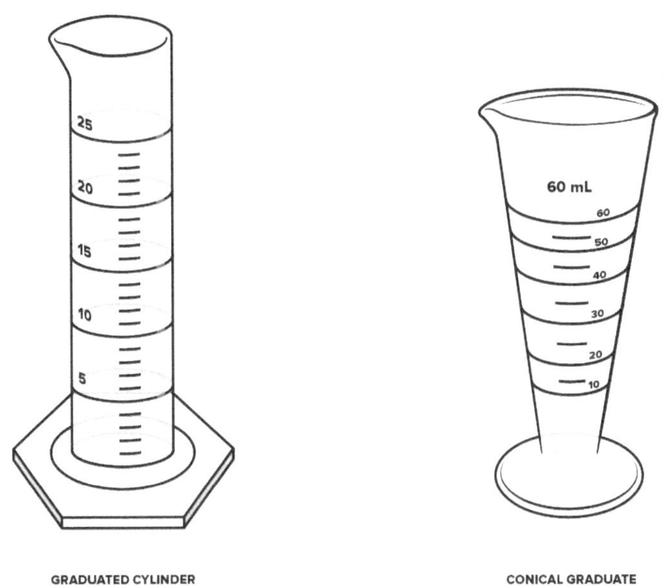
25
20
15
10
5
GRADUATED CYLINDER
60 mL
60
50
40
30
20
10
CONICAL GRADUATE

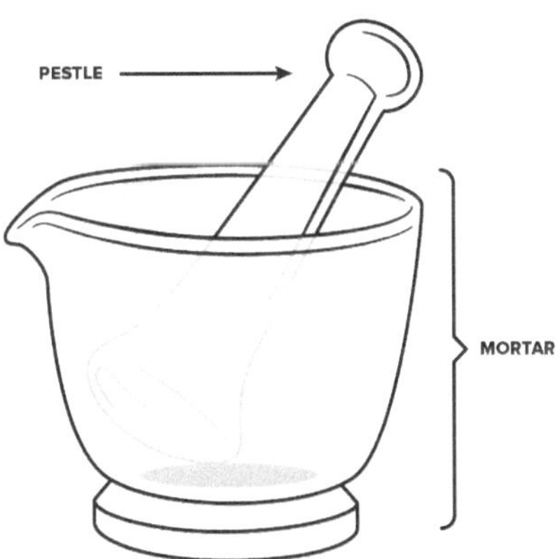
PESTLE
MORTAR

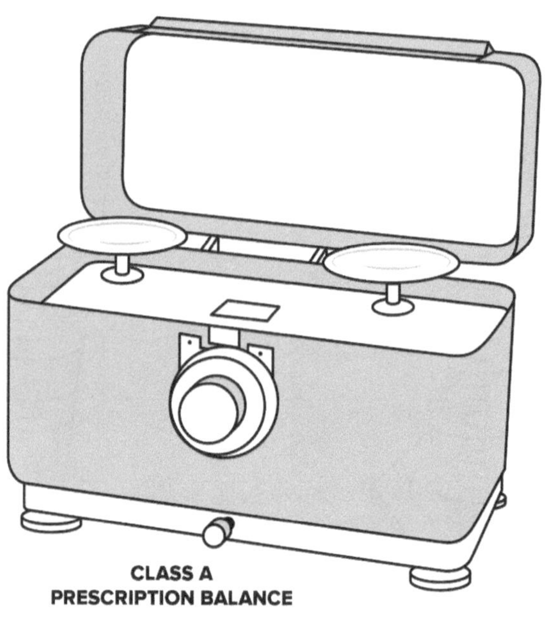

CLASS A PRESCRIPTION BALANCE

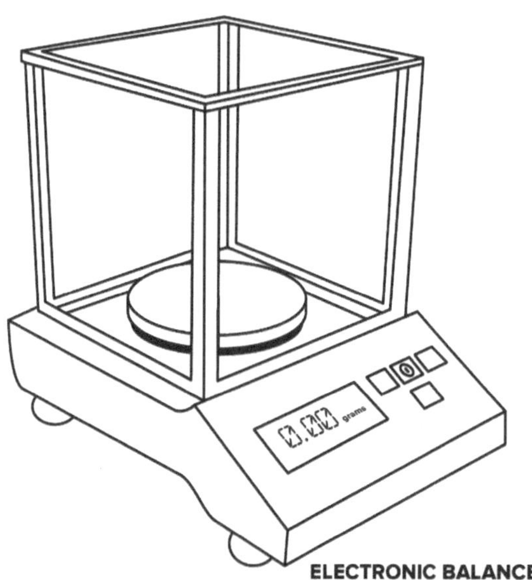

ELECTRONIC BALANCE

Note: a class A prescription balance is the standard, traditional balance used in pharmacies for measuring the weight of ingredients when compounding medications. Most pharmacists these days use an electronic balance, which is easier to use and potentially more accurate.

HOW TO MEASURE LIQUIDS

Look at the image below. If each hash mark represents one milliliter, how many milliliters of gray liquid are contained in the measuring device?

A. 32 mL
B. 31 mL
C. 30 mL
D. 29 mL

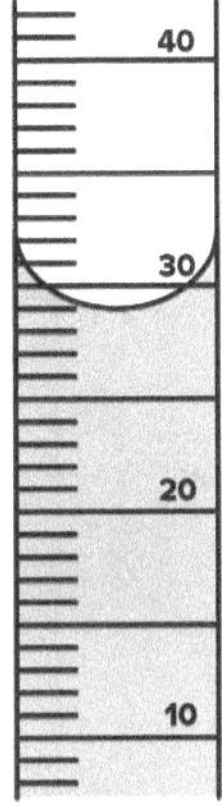

See following page for answer and explanation.

Answer: D. 29 mL

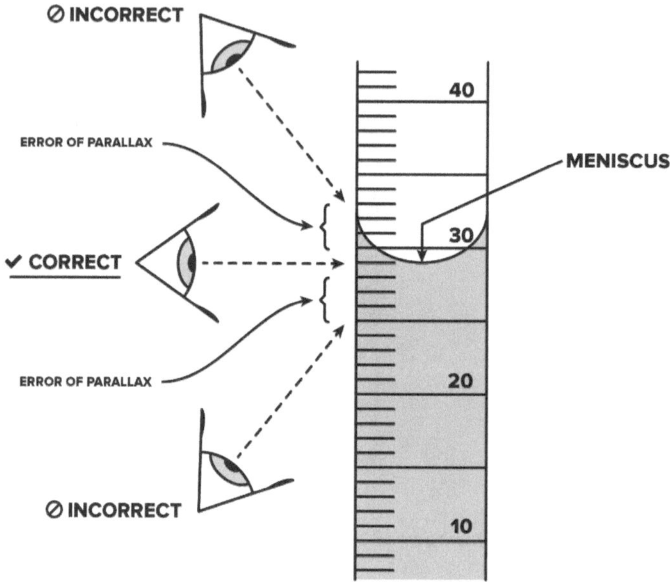

There is only one correct way to measure a liquid using a liquid measuring device, and that is *at the bottom of the meniscus* (the curve at the surface of the liquid) and *at eye level*. When measurements are made above or below eye level, the difference between the actual level and the apparent level is called the "error of parallax."

PERCENT CONCENTRATIONS

Weight/Weight % (w/w) = # of grams of API* per 100 grams of preparation.

Example

AndroGel® 1% gel contains 1 g testosterone per 100 grams of gel.

Practice Problem

How many milligrams of testosterone are contained in one 5-gram packet of AndroGel® 1% gel?

$$\frac{1 \text{ g of testosterone}}{100 \text{ g of gel}} \times \frac{5 \text{ g of gel}}{1} \times \frac{1{,}000 \text{ mg}}{\text{g}} = 50 \text{ mg of testosterone}$$

Weight/Volume % (w/v) = # of grams of API* per 100 mL of preparation.

Example

Clindamycin 1% topical solution contains 1 g clindamycin per 100 mL of solution.

Practice Problem

What is the percent concentration (w/v) of a 250-mL solution that contains 35 mg of an active ingredient?

$$\frac{0.035 \text{ g}}{250 \text{ mL}} = \frac{x}{100 \text{ mL}} \quad \therefore \quad x = \frac{0.035 \text{ g} \times 100 \text{ mL}}{250 \text{ mL}} = 0.014 \text{ g}$$

0.014 g per 100 mL = 0.014% (w/v)

Volume/Volume % (v/v) = # of mL of API* per 100 mL of preparation.

Example

Cheratussin® AC contains 3.8% (v/v) alcohol, meaning that there are 3.8-mL of alcohol in every 100-mL of Cheratussin® AC.

Practice Problem

What is the percent concentration (v/v) of a 15-mL bottle of a solution that contains 0.75-mL tea tree oil in sterile water?

$$\frac{0.75 \text{ mL of API}}{15 \text{ mL}} = \frac{x}{100 \text{ mL}} \quad \therefore \quad \frac{0.75 \text{ mL of API} \times 100 \text{ mL}}{15 \text{ mL}} = 5 \text{ mL}$$

5 mL per 100 mL=5% (v/v)

Note: API = active pharmaceutical ingredient

When expressing a concentration as a percent, why is it necessary to specify whether the concentration is in terms of w/w, w/v, or v/v?
It is necessary to specify because some substances can only be measured feasibly by weight (solids) and some substances are easier to measure by volume (liquids). Weight and volume are not equal (e.g. 1 mL of alcohol weighs 0.79 grams), except in the case of water (1 mL of water weighs 1 gram). This is because different substances have different densities (see section titled "Density and Specific Gravity" for more details on density).

PRACTICE PROBLEMS

1. A 6-month-old female is given one-half dropperful of Sodium Fluoride 0.11% (w/v) drops. How many milligrams of Sodium Fluoride did she receive?
Note: 1 dropperful = 1 mL

2. Clobetasol propionate topical solution comes in a 50-mL bottle. If each mL of solution contains 0.5 mg of clobetasol propionate, what is the percent concentration of the solution?

3. Prednisolone 15 mg/5 mL oral solution contains 5% (v/v) alcohol. How many milliliters of alcohol are there in one teaspoonful of solution?

4. Antipyrine and benzocaine otic solution contains 1.4% (w/v) benzocaine and 5.4% (w/v) antipyrine in an anhydrous glycerin base. How many milligrams of each active ingredient are present in one 15-mL bottle?

PRACTICE PROBLEM ANSWERS

1. 0.55 mg Sodium Fluoride
2. 0.05% (w/v)
3. 0.25 mL alcohol
4. 810 mg of antipyrine & 210 mg of benzocaine

RATIOS

In pharmacy, ratios are used in:
1. Compounding recipes.
2. Expressing the concentration of a liquid medication.

Ratios Used in Compounding Recipes
When used in a compounding recipe, ratios describe how many parts of each substance make up the whole. For instance, a 24-ounce cherry pie recipe that calls for a 1:1 ratio of pie dough to cherry filling would be composed of 12 ounces of pie dough and 12 ounces of cherry filling.

An order for a compounded medication will include (at minimum) this basic information:
1. The names of each ingredient.
2. The amount or ratio of each ingredient.
3. The amount of final product desired.*

* In some cases, the amount of final product desired may be written by the prescriber as "QS," which comes from the Latin phrase "quantum sufficit" meaning "as much as suffices." In these cases, you will need to calculate how much to prepare based on the dosing instructions. See the following example.

EXAMPLE PROBLEM

What volume of each ingredient will you need to compound the following prescription?

James Smith, D.O.
Simplified Medical Clinic
10001 N. Main St. Suite 100A, Simple City, USA 24680
Telephone# 123-555-1234

Name George Simpleton Age 50
Address 222 North Main St. Simple City, USA 24680 Date 1/14/16

Rx

1 Part Viscous Lidocaine : 2 Parts Diphenhydramine 12.5 mg/5 mL Elixir
Dispense QS
Swish and swallow 3 tsp QID x 14 days

(NR) 1 2 3 4 5 PRN

James Smith, D.O.

Prescriber must write 'Brand Medically Necessary' on the prescription to prohibit generic substitution.

Solution:

Step 1: Since the quantity is written as QS, you must calculate the amount of final product desired. This is easy, because you know how much product is being used in one dose (3 teaspoonsful), you know how many doses the patient will take each day (4 doses/day), and you know how long the patient will be taking the medication (14 days).

$$\frac{15 \text{ mL}}{\text{dose}} \times \frac{4 \text{ doses}}{\text{day}} \times \frac{14 \text{ days}}{1} = 840 \text{ mL}$$

Step 2: Calculate the amount that makes up 1 part of the 3 part mixture by dividing the amount of final product desired by 3 parts.

$$\frac{840 \text{ mL}}{3 \text{ parts}} = 280 \text{ mL/part}$$

Step 3: Now that you know the amount that represents 1 part, calculate the amount of each ingredient that will be needed to compound the prescription.

$$\frac{1 \text{ part of Lidocaine } 2\%}{1} \times \frac{280 \text{ mL}}{\text{part}} = 280 \text{ mL of Lidocaine } 2\%$$

$$\frac{2 \text{ parts Diphenhydramine } 12.5/5 \text{ mL}}{1} \times \frac{280 \text{ mL}}{\text{part}} = 560 \text{ mL Diphenhydramine } 12.5 \text{ mg/5 mL}$$

Answer: 280 mL Lidocaine 2% & 560 mL diphenhydramine 12.5 mg/5 mL

Ratios Used to Express the Concentration of a Medication

When used to express a concentration, a ratio describes how many parts of the active ingredient are present in a certain number of parts of the total formulation. For example, epinephrine 1:10,000 solution contains one part epinephrine in 10,000 parts of solution. The conversion factors below are for your reference.

CONVERSION FACTORS FOR CONCENTRATIONS EXPRESSED BY A RATIO
1:1 = 1 gram per mL = 1 g/mL
1:1,000 = 1 x 10^{-3} grams per mL = 1 mg/mL
1:1,000,000 = 1 x 10^{-6} grams per mL = 1 mcg/mL

EXAMPLE PROBLEM

How many milligrams of epinephrine are there in 2 milliliters of Epinephrine 1:1,000,000 solution?

Solution:

Step 1: Convert the ratio into a value with metric units using the conversion factor above.

According to conversion factor above, 1:1,000,000 = 1 mcg/mL

Step 2: Apply the following equation **or** use the unit conversion/proportion approach.

$$\frac{\text{Weight}_1}{\text{Volume}_1} = \frac{\text{Weight}_2}{\text{Volume}_2}$$

Insert the given information into the equation.
Weigth $_1$ = 1 mcg
Volume $_1$ = 1 mL
Weight $_2$ = ?
Volume $_2$ = 2 mL

$$\frac{1\text{ mcg}}{1\text{ mL}} = \frac{\text{Weight}_2}{2\text{ mL}}$$

Step 3: Get the unknown value (Weight_2) alone.

$$\text{Weight}_2 = \frac{1\text{ mcg x } 2\text{ mL}}{1\text{ mL}} = 2\text{ mcg}$$

Answer: 2 mcg

PRACTICE PROBLEMS

1. The package for EpiPen Jr 2-Pak® comes with 2 Auto-Injectors, each one containing 0.3 mL of a 1:2000 epinephrine solution. How many milligrams of epinephrine are in one EpiPen Jr 2-Pak®?

2. What is the ratio strength of a 20-mL solution that contains 200 mcg of drug?

3. What is the ratio strength of a solution that contains 1 mg of drug per mL of solution?

4. How many milliliters of a 1:200 stock solution of Lidocaine would be required to compound a prescription for 50 mL of 0.25% Lidocaine solution?

5. If you have 1 gallon of a 1:40 solution of Drug XYZ, how many Liters of 1:1,000 solution of Drug XYZ can you compound?

PRACTICE PROBLEM ANSWERS

1. 0.3 mg (0.15 mg of epinephrine per Auto-Injector, and there are two Auto-Injectors in one EpiPen Jr 2-Pak®)
2. 1:10,000
3. 1:1,000
4. 25 mL
5. 94.6 L

CALCULATIONS USED IN COMPOUNDING

Alligation is a great way to solve certain compounding math problems. Use alligation when you are given two products with different concentrations of the same drug and you need a concentration that falls somewhere in the between (or when you have a higher concentration than what is desired and you want to dilute it with an inert substance like water or petrolatum). Start by drawing an X with a hollow center.

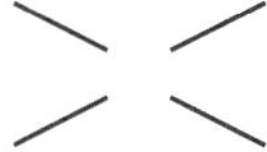

In every alligation problem, you will have to compound a prescription for a certain concentration using two products. One product will have a higher-than-desired concentration, and the other product will have a lower-than-desired concentration. For example, let's say we have a 1% cream of Product B and a 10% cream of Product B, and we want to make a cream that contains 3% Product B. Write the value for the high concentration product at the top left, and write the value for the low concentration product at the bottom left.

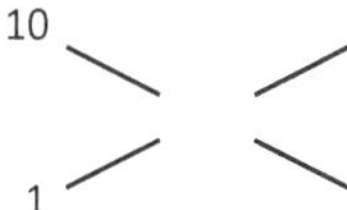

Next, write the value of the desired concentration in the center.

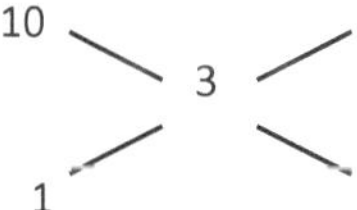

Then calculate the difference between the numbers on the left side of the X and the number at the center. Write the answer, following the diagonal line, at the opposite corner of the X.

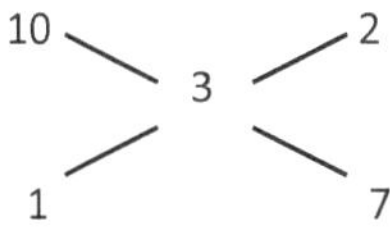

The numbers on the right side of the X indicate the proportion of each ingredient needed to compound a formulation of the desired concentration.

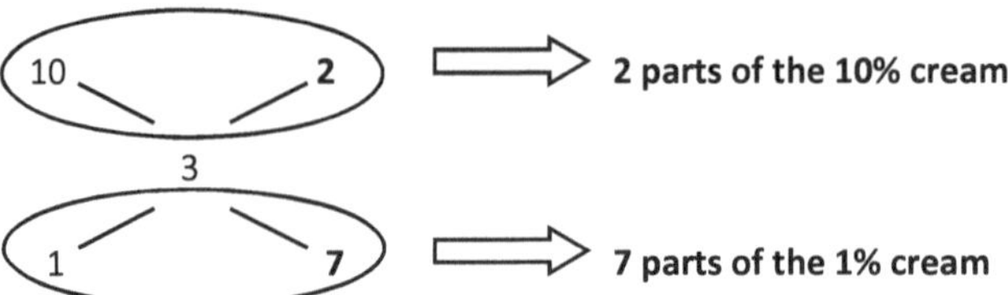

At this point, you would have all the information needed to solve the problem. Let's say the prescription called for 60 grams of 3% Product B cream. Based on the results of the alligation, you know that the cream would be made up of nine equal parts (2 parts of 10% cream and 7 parts of 1% cream). Divide 60 grams into nine equal parts (60 g ÷ 9 parts = 6.67 g/part). You would need 13.3 g (6.67 g/part x 2 parts = 13.3 g) of 10% cream and 46.7 g (6.67 g/part x 7 parts = 46.7 g) of 1% cream to compound 60 g of 3 % Product B cream. Now, practice as many of these as you can!

EXAMPLE PROBLEMS

You need 30 g of Triamcinolone 0.05% ointment, but all you have in stock is Triamcinolone 0.025% and 0.1% ointment. How much of each ingredient will you need in order to compound this prescription?

Solution:

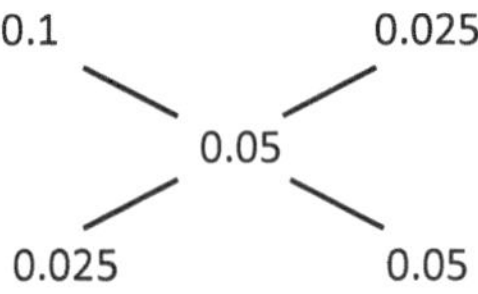

0.025 : 0.05 = 1 : 2

1 part of 0.1% triamcinolone : 2 parts of 0.025% triamcinolone

$$\frac{30\text{ g}}{3\text{ parts}} \times \frac{1\text{ part of }0.1\%\text{ triamcinolone}}{1} = 10\text{ g of }0.1\%\text{ triamcinolone}$$

$$\frac{30\text{ g}}{3\text{ parts}} \times \frac{2\text{ parts of }0.025\%\text{ triamcinolone}}{1} = 20\text{ g of }0.025\%\text{ triamcinolone}$$

Answer: 10 g of 0.1% and 20 g of 0.025% triamcinolone ointment

You have 800 mL of 70% alcohol solution. How much water will you need to add in order to make a 10% alcohol solution?
Note: Assume the water contains 0% alcohol.

Solution:

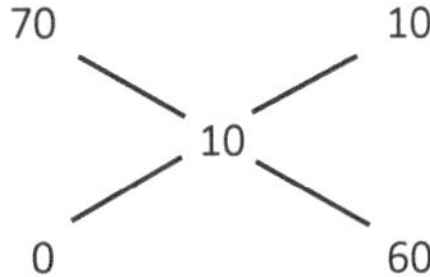

$$10 \text{ parts} = 800 \text{ mL} \therefore 1 \text{ part} = 80 \text{ mL}$$

$$60 \text{ parts} \times \frac{80 \text{ mL}}{\text{part}} = 4{,}800 \text{ mL}$$

Answer: 4,800 mL of water

How many grams of pure Sodium Chloride must be added to 10 mL of normal saline solution to create a 3% NaCl solution?
Note: Pure NaCl is 100% NaCl.

Solution:

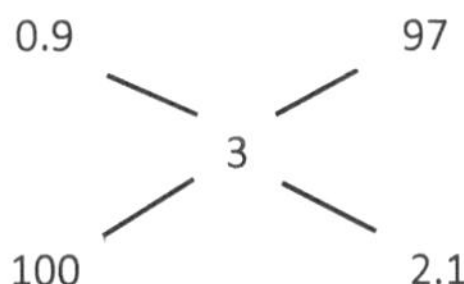

$$97 \text{ parts of } 0.9\% \text{ NaCl} = 10 \text{ mL} \therefore 1 \text{ part} = \frac{10 \text{ mL}}{97} = 0.103 \text{ mL}$$

$$2.1 \text{ parts} \times \frac{0.103 \text{ mL}}{\text{part}} = 0.22 \text{ mL} \sim 0.22 \text{ g}$$

Answer: 0.22 g of pure NaCl

You need to compound an IV solution of 2.5 mg/mL Vancomycin in D5W using a vial that contains 1 gram of Vancomycin in 20 mL. How much D5W will be needed?

Solution:

Step 1: Convert the concentrations to percentages.

Note: A one-percent solution contains one gram per one hundred milliliters (1% = 1 g/100 mL). Knowing this, you can convert the given units to a percentage by calculating the number of grams in 100 mL.

Desired Concentration (To Be Compounded)

$$\frac{2.5 \text{ mg}}{\text{mL}} \times \frac{1 \text{ g}}{1{,}000 \text{ mg}} \times 100 \text{ mL} = 0.25 \text{ g}$$

If 100 mL of the solution contains 0.25 g of Vancomycin, then the percent concentration would be 0.25%.

Given Concentration (In Vial)

$$\frac{1 \text{ g}}{20 \text{ mL}} \times 5 = \frac{5 \text{ g}}{100 \text{ mL}} = 5\%$$

To summarize, we are given a 5% Vancomycin solution, and we want to create a 0.25% Vancomycin solution using D5W (contains 0% Vancomycin).

Step 2: Alligation math.

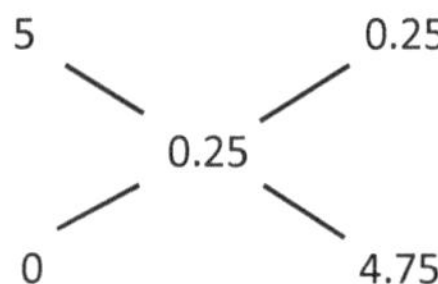

0.25 parts of 5% Vancomycin : 4.75 parts of D5W

In other words (if you multiply each part by a factor of 4), the compound must be made up of 1 part of 5% Vancomycin and 19 parts D5W.

We know we are using 20 mL of the 5% Vancomycin solution, so:

1 part = 20 mL ∴ 19 parts = 19 x 20 mL = 380 mL

Answer: 380 mL of D5W

PRACTICE PROBLEMS

1. How much of each ingredient will be needed to make 50 mL of 1% KCl solution from 3% KCl solution and water?

2. How many Liters of 3% H_2O_2 and 6% H_2O_2 will you need to mix together to make 2 Liters of 4.5% H_2O_2?

3. You need to dilute a 5% Lidocaine cream to compound 45 grams of 4% Lidocaine cream using a cream base. How much 5% Lidocaine cream will be needed to compound this prescription?

4. How many grams of 1% Hydrocortisone cream will need to be mixed with 100% Hydrocortisone powder to make 2 ounces of 2.5% Hydrocortisone cream?
Note: 1 ounce = 28.35 grams

PRACTICE PROBLEM ANSWERS

1. 16.7 mL of 3% KCl solution; 33.3 mL of water
2. 1 Liter of 3% H_2O_2 & 1 Liter of 6% H_2O_2
3. 36 grams of 5% Lidocaine cream
4. 55.8 grams of 1% Hydrocortisone cream

Which chapter of the USP Compounding Compendium provides guidance on good compounding practices in preparing non-sterile compounded drug products?
USP Chapter 795.

What is a diluent?
A diluent is an inactive product used to dilute an active pharmaceutical ingredient.

What is trituration?
Trituration is the process of reducing the particle size of a powder, usually by use of a mortar and pestle.

What is "sensitivity requirement?"
The sensitivity requirement is the mass needed to move the balance marker by one space (see the illustration below). For a class A prescription balance, the sensitivity requirement is 6 mg.

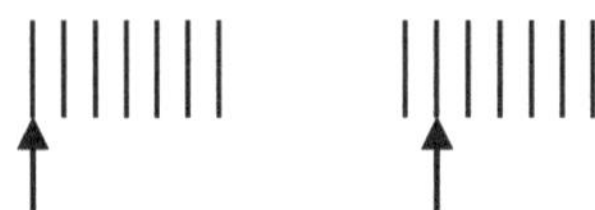

What is geometric dilution?
Geometric dilution is the process of expanding the weight of the active pharmaceutical ingredient by adding an inert substance (i.e. diluent) in a fashion that yields a homogeneous mixture. In more simplified terms, you dilute the active ingredient and mix it well to ensure even mixture.

What is the purpose of geometric dilution?
Many drug doses are very small (in the microgram to milligram range). Accurately measuring these small doses can be difficult. To obtain an accurate measurement, you have two options: 1) use a highly sensitive analytical balance or 2) dilute the drug to make it weigh more. The standard pharmacy balance is a class A prescription balance. This type of balance is sensitive enough to measure 120 mg or more within 5% error. To accurately measure smaller quantities with a class A prescription balance, you must dilute the drug.

For example...
If you want to measure 60 mg of a drug using a class A prescription balance, you could take 120 mg (the lowest quantity that can be accurately measured with this type of balance) of the pure (100%) drug powder and mix it with 120 mg of lactose (an inert substance; diluent). Now you have a powder that is 50% drug and 50% lactose. Now you can measure 120 mg of this mixture to obtain 60 mg of drug. The trick is to never use the balance to measure any quantity less than 120 mg. If you do, you will not stay within the 5% error requirement (to gain a better understanding of percent error, refer to the section on non-sterile compounding).

How do you perform geometric dilution?
Take the active pharmaceutical ingredient and add an equal amount of diluent. Triturate the mixture until you are convinced it is homogeneous. Then add an equal amount of diluent to the mixture and triturate as before. Repeat the steps until all of the ingredients form an even mixture.

ILLUSTRATED EXAMPLE OF GEOMETRIC DILUTION

Dilute 200 mg of amlodipine powder with 1,400 mg of lactose powder to create a homogeneous mixture with a total mass of 1,600 mg.

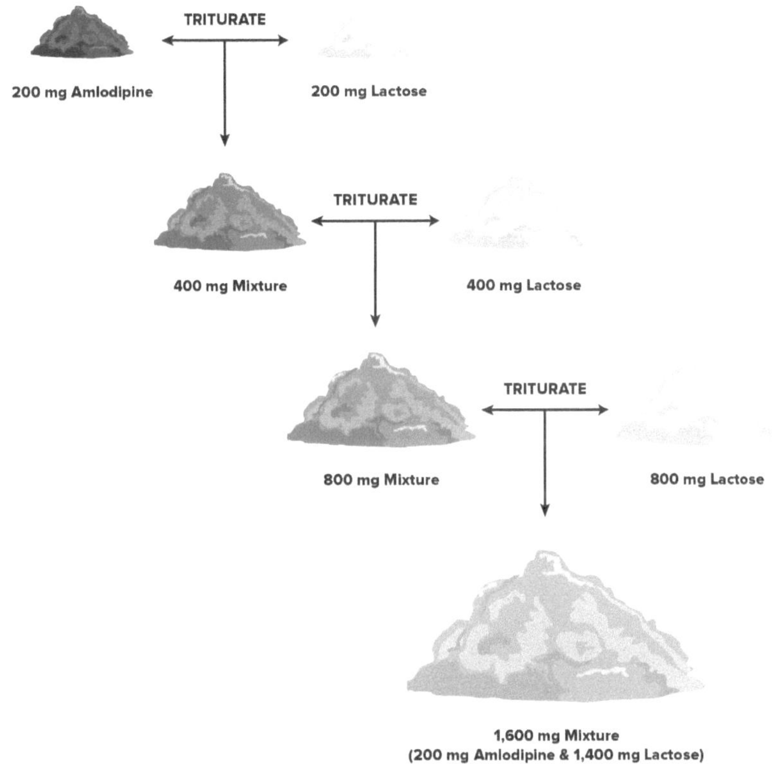

Key Point: If you were to triturate 200 mg of amlodipine with 1,400 mg of lactose all at once, you would probably achieve an uneven (heterogeneous) mixture. By slowly adding the diluent in this stepwise fashion, you greatly increase the likelihood of achieving an even (homogeneous) mixture.

What is the percent error (% error)?
Percent error refers to the accuracy of a measurement. For instance, 5% error means that the measurement is within +/- 5% of the actual value. In pharmacy, the highest acceptable percent error is usually 5% but can be even less in some cases.

How are the "sensitivity requirement" and "percent error" related?
These terms are related according to the following equation:

$$\% \text{ Error} = \frac{\text{Sensitivity Requirement}}{\text{Desired Weight}} \times 100\%$$

EXAMPLE PROBLEMS

Given that the sensitivity requirement of a class A prescription balance is 6 mg, what is the minimum quantity that can be weighed within 5% error?

Solution:

This problem can be solved using the above equation. The terms were re-written to reflect the nature of this specific question.
Note: LWQ = least weighable quantity.

$$\text{Maximum Acceptable \% Error} = \frac{\text{Sensitivity Requirement}}{\text{LWQ}} \times 100\%$$

$$5\% = \frac{6 \text{ mg}}{\text{LWQ}} \times 100\%$$

Rearrange the equation to solve for LWQ...

$$\text{LWQ} = \frac{6 \text{ mg}}{5\%} \times 100\% = 120 \text{ mg}$$

Answer: 120 mg

If you were using a class A prescription balance to measure 20 mg of Powder X, what would the percent error be?

Solution:

$$\% \text{ Error} = \frac{\text{Sensitivity Requirement}}{\text{Desired Weight}} \times 100\% = \frac{6 \text{ mg}}{20 \text{ mg}} \times 100\% = 30\%$$

Answer: 30% error

Is this an acceptable level of error?
No, the highest acceptable level of error is 5%.

If you needed to measure 20 mg of a Powder X using a class A prescription balance, how would you do it while achieving a percent error ≤ 5%?
Take 120 mg of the substance (which can be measured within 5% error) and use geometric dilution to create a homogeneous mixture of 1 part (120 mg) Powder X and 5 parts (600 mg) diluent (e.g. lactose). Then, using the class A prescription balance, measure out 120 mg of the mixture, which will contain 20 mg of Powder X.

You are compounding a prescription which requires you to measure 40 mL of a liquid. Which of the following pieces of equipment should you use?

A. 10 mL graduated cylinder
B. 50 ml graduated cylinder
C. 20 mL syringe
D. 60 mL syringe

Answer: B. 50 mL graduated cylinder

EQUIPMENT SELECTION TIP

Use the smallest measuring device that will hold the desired volume.

PRACTICE PROBLEMS

1. You want to measure 10 mg of a substance within 1% error without diluting it. The sensitivity requirement of your balance would need to be ___.

2. You are using a class A prescription balance to measure 9 grams of maltose. What percent error will you get with this measurement?

3. You want to measure out 20 mg of hydrocortisone within 5% error using a class A prescription balance. Since the LWQ (least weighable quantity) is 120 mg, you know you will have to perform a geometric dilution to obtain a 20 mg measurement within 5% error. How much diluent powder and hydrocortisone will need to be combined to perform the geometric dilution?

4. After completing the geometric dilution from *practice problem 3* (above), what is the ratio of hydrocortisone to diluent powder?

5. From practice problem 3, what is the percent concentration of hydrocortisone in the resulting powder mixture?

6. From practice problem 3, what is the fraction of hydrocortisone in the resulting powder mixture?

PRACTICE PROBLEM ANSWERS

1) 0.1 mg
2) 0.067%
3) 600 mg of diluent powder & 120 mg of hydrocortisone
4) 1:5 hydrocortisone to diluent powder
5) 16.67%
6) 1/6

CALCULATING DAYS' SUPPLY

When insurance companies are billed for prescriptions, the pharmacy technician and pharmacist are responsible for calculating the days' supply being dispensed. If you bill an insurance company for a days' supply less than that actually dispensed (e.g. dispense a 30-day supply of medication and bill the insurance as though it were a 10-day supply) the insurance company can issue a "charge-back" during an audit (i.e. the pharmacy would have to pay the insurance company back; may also be referred to as "recoupment" by insurance companies). The most commonly prescribed medications are available from the manufacturer in the form of tablets or capsules ("solid oral dosage forms"). In these cases, determining the days' supply is a simple one-step calculation.

EXAMPLE PROBLEMS

What is the days' supply for a prescription of 30 tablets of Drug X with the instructions to take one tablet by mouth once daily?

$$\frac{30 \text{ tablets}}{1} \times \frac{\text{day}}{1 \text{ tablet}} = 30 \text{ days}$$

What is the days' supply for a prescription of 60 tablets of Drug AB9012 with the instructions to take one tablet three times daily as needed for pain?

$$\frac{60 \text{ tablets}}{1} \times \frac{\text{day}}{3 \text{ tablets}} = 20 \text{ days}$$

Note: When the instructions include the term "as needed," assume the patient will use the maximum amount when calculating the days' supply.

Calculating the days' supply of a non-solid dosage form (e.g. oral liquids, eye drops, ear drops, nasal sprays, and inhalers) can be more challenging. Study the example problems on the next two pages, then practice these calculations yourself until you master them!

USE THE FOLLOWING INFORMATION TO COMPLETE THE PROBLEMS IN THIS SECTION:

ProAir®, Proventil®, and Ventolin® each contain 120 puffs/inhaler
Astepro® nasal spray contains 200 sprays/bottle
Flonase® nasal spray contains 120 sprays/bottle
Xalatan® eye drops contain 2.5 mL/bottle

MORE EXAMPLE PROBLEMS

How many days will a 4-ounce bottle of cetirizine 5 mg/5 mL solution last if the instructions are to take one-half teaspoonful QHS?
Note: Make sure you read the question carefully!

$$\frac{120 \text{ mL}}{\text{bottle}} \times \frac{\text{tsp}}{5 \text{ mL}} \times \frac{\text{day}}{0.5 \text{ tsp}} = 48 \text{ days/bottle}$$

What would the days' supply be on a prescription for Flonase® nasal spray if the instructions are 1 spray in each nostril QD?

$$\frac{120 \text{ sprays}}{\text{bottle}} \times \frac{\text{day}}{2 \text{ sprays}} = 60 \text{ days/bottle}$$

Try it yourself: **Calculate the days' supply of 1 bottle of Astepro® if the instructions say to instill 1 spray into each nostril BID.**

Answer: 50-day supply

A prescription is written for 3 Ventolin® HFA Inhalers with the instructions to inhale 2 puffs PO Q4-6H PRN wheezing. Each inhaler contains enough medication for 200 puffs. What would the days' supply of this prescription be?

$$\frac{3 \text{ inhalers}}{1} \times \frac{200 \text{ puffs}}{\text{inhaler}} \times \frac{\text{day}}{12 \text{ puffs}} = 50 \text{ days}$$

TEST YOUR KNOWLEDGE

How many drops are in one milliliter (1 mL)?

Between 15 and 20 drops.

Note: In general, you should calculate days' supply based on 20 drops/mL.

What is the days' supply for a 7.5 mL bottle of Ciprodex® Otic Solution with the instructions: ii gtts AS QID until gone?

A. 7 days
B. 10 days
C. 12 days
D. 19 days
E. 25 days

Solution:

Step 1: Interpret the sig.

"ii gtts AS QID until gone"
= instill two drops into the left ear four times daily until gone.

Step 2: Since the question does not specify how many drops are in one milliliter, calculate the days' supply based on the conversion factor of 20 drops/mL.

$$\frac{7.5 \text{ mL}}{1} \times \frac{20 \text{ drops}}{\text{mL}} \times \frac{\text{day}}{8 \text{ drops}} = 18.75 \text{ days} \therefore 19 \text{ days}$$

Answer: D. 19 days

You are dispensing a 5-mL bottle of ciprofloxacin 0.3% ophthalmic solution with instructions to instill two drops into each eye three times daily until gone. What is the days' supply of this prescription (assume 20 drops/mL)?

$$\frac{5 \text{ mL}}{1} \times \frac{20 \text{ drops}}{\text{mL}} \times \frac{\text{day}}{12 \text{ drops}} = 8 \text{ days}$$

THE RULE OF HAND

One (1) gram of topical medication is roughly enough to cover one side (palm and fingers) of four flat hands. Use the Rule of Hand when calculating the days' supply of topical medications.

PRACTICE PROBLEMS

1. What is the days' supply for a 15-gram tube of acne medication with instructions to apply to the entire face nightly?
Note: The area of the face is roughly equal to the area of two flat hands

2. You are dispensing two Ventolin® HFA inhalers with instructions for the patient to inhale one to two puffs by mouth every four to six hours as needed for shortness of breath. What will the days' supply be for this prescription?

3. What is the days' supply for a quantity of 60 venlafaxine ER 37.5 mg capsules with the following instructions: i PO QD x 7 days, then i PO BID x 7 days, then ii QAM and i QPM thereafter?

4. What is the days' supply for a 120-mL bottle of Tussionex® suspension with the following instructions: take i tsp PO up to TID PRN for cough?

5. You dispense a prescription for methotrexate 2.5 mg tablets with instructions to take three tablets by mouth weekly. What is the days' supply for 30 tablets?

6. NovoLog® FlexPen is available in a package that contains five pens. Each pen contains three milliliters of NovoLog® insulin. If a patient uses 11 units SQ every morning and 9 units SQ every evening with a meal, what is the days' supply for a single package that contains five pens?
(**Note:** the concentration of NovoLog® insulin is 100 units per milliliter)

7. Antipyrine-benzocaine otic solution comes in a 15-mL bottle. What is the days' supply if the instructions are as follows: instill 2-4 gtts AU up to QID PRN?
(**Note:** Assume there are 20 drops per mL)

PRACTICE PROBLEM ANSWERS

1. 30 days
2. 33 days
3. 27 days
4. 8 days
5. 70 days
6. 75 days
7. 9 days

"STEROID TAPER"... WHAT DOES IT MEAN?

The human body naturally produces steroid hormones. Taking steroids medicinally leads to a reduction in the body's internal production of steroids. At high doses, use of medicinal steroids can shut down steroid hormone production within the body entirely. For this reason, when discontinuing high doses of steroids, it is necessary to decrease the dose gradually over time (as opposed to abruptly stopping the medication) to give the body time to turn steroid production back on. This process of gradual reduction is called a taper.

When doctors prescribe short courses of a high-dose steroid, they will often use a dose pack. An example of a steroid dose pack is the prednisone 10 mg 6-day dose pack where the patient takes 6 tablets the first day and decreases by one tablet daily until finished (6, 5, 4, 3, 2, 1, stop). With dose packs, the manufacturer includes the instructions directly on the packaging. This makes it more convenient for the patient and the prescriber.

It should be noted that steroid tapers can be accomplished without the use of a dose pack. For instance, a prescriber could issue a prescription for prednisone with instructions to take 30 mg daily for 3 days, 20 mg daily for 3 days, 10 mg daily for 3 days, 5 mg daily for 3 days, and then stop.

Note: The term "taper" can also be used to describe gradually increasing the dose of a medication (also known as "titrating" the dose). Starting at a low dose and increasing it slowly up to the optimal therapeutic dose allows the body to gradually build a tolerance to the drug, thus reducing the incidence of side effects. For example, gabapentin is often initiated at a low dose and then gradually increased to a more effective dose in an attempt to avoid the side effect of drowsiness. Another example is metformin, which is usually dosed in a similar fahion to avoid side effects such as upset stomach and diarrhea.

When dealing with tapers, days' supply calculations can be more challenging. Remember, when an insurance company is improperly billed for a prescription, they can recoup previously paid money in an audit; in other words, the pharmacy must pay them back. For instance, if an insurance company audits your pharmacy and finds that a prescription was dispensed for a 90-day supply, but you billed them as though the prescription were only a 30-day supply, the insurance company can say that the claim was not submitted correctly and demand that the pharmacy pay them back.

Useful Fact: Prednisone dose packs come in two sizes: a 48-tablet 6-day dose pack or a 21-tablet 12-day dose pack.

While we are on the topic, let's talk about the term "dosepak." Some people use the terms "dosepak" and "dose pack" interchangeably. Truth be told, "dosepak" is not a real word; rather, it is a portion of one of Pfizer's brand name drugs, the Medrol® Dosepak™. The name is similar to one of Pfizer's other inventions, the Z-pak®. The names ending in "pak" belong to Pfizer. All other dose packs (such as prednisone dose packs, generic methylprednisolone dose packs, and generic azithromycin dose packs) are just called "dose packs."

CALCULATING DOSES BASED ON WEIGHT

Weight-based dosing always requires the patient's weight to be in units of kilograms (kg). Here in the United States, we typically measure a person's weight in terms of pounds, not kilograms. For this reason, converting a patient's weight from pounds to kilograms will usually be the first step in calculating a weight-based dose. A lot of scenarios involve converting a patient's weight from pounds to kilograms, so it is extremely important that you master this calculation. Fortunately, the calculation is simple. Just remember that 1 kg = 2.2 lbs, and get a lot of practice by working through the examples and practice problems.

EXAMPLE PROBLEMS

Infliximab is prescribed to a patient at the dose of 5 mg/kg. The patient weighs 154 pounds. How many milligrams of infliximab should be dispensed as one dose?

$$\frac{154 \text{ lb}}{1} \times \frac{1 \text{ kg}}{2.2 \text{ lb}} \times \frac{5 \text{ mg}}{\text{kg}} = 350 \text{ mg}$$

You calculate the appropriate dose of infliximab to be 350 mg. The dose is going to be administered IV in 250 mL of 0.9% NaCl. Infliximab comes in a vial containing 100 mg/20 mL solution. How many vials will you need to open in order to fill this prescription?

Answer: 4 vials (you will only use 3.5 vials-worth of the drug, but you will need to open 4 vials since you cannot open half of a vial)

How many milliliters of the drug solution will be needed to obtain 350 mg of infliximab for the aforementioned prescription?

$$\frac{350 \text{ mg}}{1} \times \frac{20 \text{ mL}}{100 \text{ mg}} = 70 \text{ mL}$$

Vancomycin is being dosed at 15 mg/kg for a patient that weighs 241 pounds and has a fever. How many milliliters of vancomycin 1 gram/20 mL solution will be needed to compound this prescription?

$$\frac{241 \text{ lb}}{1} \times \frac{1 \text{ kg}}{2.2 \text{ lb}} \times \frac{15 \text{ mg}}{\text{kg}} \times \frac{20 \text{ mL}}{1 \text{ g}} \times \frac{1 \text{ g}}{1{,}000 \text{ mg}} = 32.9 \text{ mL}$$

Note: Frequently you will receive problems that contain irrelevant information (in this case, the fact that the patient has a fever). Don't be distracted by this type of information; just move on and solve the problem using the relevant information.

CALCULATING DOSES BASED ON BODY SURFACE AREA (BSA)

FORMULA FOR BODY SURFACE AREA (BSA)

$$\text{BSA} = \sqrt{\frac{\text{height (cm) x weight (kg)}}{3{,}600}}$$

Note: Cancer chemotherapy drug dosing is commonly based on body surface area.

EXAMPLE PROBLEMS

What is the BSA of a patient that is 5 feet and 4 inches tall and weighs 110 pounds?

$$\sqrt{\frac{64 \text{ in}}{1} \times \frac{2.54 \text{ cm}}{\text{in}} \times \frac{110 \text{ lb}}{1} \times \frac{1 \text{ kg}}{2.2 \text{ lb}} \times \frac{1}{3{,}600}} = 1.50 \text{ m}^2$$

Note: BSA is expressed in units of square meters (m^2).

The appropriate dose of Doxorubicin is 550 mg/m^2. How many milligrams are required to provide three doses to a male patient 6' 1" tall weighing 225 lbs?

$$\frac{73 \text{ in}}{1} \times \frac{2.54 \text{ cm}}{\text{in}} = 185 \text{ cm}$$

$$\frac{225 \text{ lb}}{1} \times \frac{1 \text{ kg}}{2.2 \text{ lb}} = 102 \text{ kg}$$

$$\sqrt{\frac{185 \text{ cm x } 102 \text{ kg}}{3{,}600}} \times \frac{550 \text{ mg}}{\text{m}^2} \times \frac{3 \text{ doses}}{1} = 3{,}777 \text{ mg}$$

Note: When you convert the height and weight to the metric system separately (as demonstrated above), and then plug the numbers into the equation for BSA, your final answer will be slightly less accurate due to rounding. For this reason, it is better to perform all of the calculations at the same time (see example below).

$$\left(\sqrt{\frac{73 \text{ in}}{1} \times \frac{2.54 \text{ cm}}{\text{in}} \times \frac{225 \text{ lb}}{1} \times \frac{1 \text{ kg}}{2.2 \text{ lb}} \times \frac{1}{3{,}600}}\right) \times \frac{550 \text{ mg}}{\text{m}^2} \times \frac{3}{1} = 3{,}787 \text{ mg}$$

This answer is more accurate, since the converted weight and height were not rounded.
In this case, there were only 2 significant figures, so technically the correct answer is 3,800 mg. Both approaches yield the same answer for all practical purposes; however, it is always best to use the most accurate approach when solving math problems and then round your final answer up or down as necessary.

CALCULATING PEDIATRIC DOSES

What are the three major methods for calculating pediatric doses based on adult dosing information?

1. Clark's Rule
2. Young's Rule
3. BSA dosing

CLARK'S RULE

$$\text{Child Dose} = \frac{\text{Weight (lb)}}{\text{150 lb}} \times \text{Adult Dose}$$

What is the significance of 150 pounds?
150 pounds is the average adult weight.

Note: If the child's weight is given in kilograms, you must convert the weight to pounds. To do this, multiply the kilogram weight by the conversion factor of 2.2 pounds/kilogram.

YOUNG'S RULE

$$\text{Child Dose} = \frac{\text{Age}}{(\text{Age} + 12)} \times \text{Adult Dose}$$

Note: If the child's age is given in months, you must convert or round to the nearest year!

BSA DOSING

$$\text{Child Dose} = \frac{\text{BSA}}{1.73\ \text{m}^2} \times \text{Adult Dose}$$

What is the significance of the value 1.73 m^2?
1.73 m^2 is the average adult body surface area (BSA).

Remember the equation... $\text{BSA} = \sqrt{\frac{\text{height (cm)} \times \text{weight (kg)}}{3{,}600}}$

Note: Keep an eye on those units! Height must be in centimeters and weight must be in kilograms!

EXAMPLE PROBLEMS

You are dispensing a prescription for prednisone for a 6-year-old patient that is 3′ 5″ tall and weighs 49 pounds. What is the appropriate pediatric dose for this patient based on BSA dosing if the adult dose is 20 mg?

Solution:

$$\text{Child Dose} = \frac{\left(\sqrt{\dfrac{\dfrac{41 \text{ in}}{1} \times \dfrac{2.54 \text{ cm}}{\text{in}} \times \dfrac{49 \text{ lb}}{1} \times \dfrac{\text{kg}}{2.2 \text{ lb}}}{3{,}600}}\right)}{1.73 \text{ m}^2} \times 20 \text{ mg} = 9.3 \text{ mg}$$

Answer: 9.3 mg

What is the appropriate dose based on Young's Rule?

Solution:

$$\text{Child Dose} = \frac{6}{(6 + 12)} \times 20 \text{ mg} = 6.7 \text{ mg}$$

Answer: 6.7 mg

What is the appropriate dose based on Clark's Rule?

Solution:

$$\text{Child Dose} = \frac{49 \text{ lb}}{150 \text{ lb}} \times 20 \text{ mg} = 6.5 \text{ mg}$$

Answer: 6.5 mg

Using Clark's Rule, calculate the appropriate dose of Drug X for a 30 kg child (the adult dose is 750 mg).

A. 150 mg
B. 250 mg
C. 300 mg
D. 330 mg
E. 460 mg

Solution:

$$\text{Child Dose} = \frac{\left(\frac{30\text{ kg}}{1} \times \frac{2.2\text{ lb}}{\text{kg}}\right)}{150\text{ lb}} \times 750\text{ mg} = 330\text{ mg}$$

Answer: D. 330 mg

Note: Never overlook what units you are working with. If you forget to convert the patient's weight from kilograms to pounds before using Clark's Rule, you will miss questions like this.

Practice Problems

1. The adult dose of Drug HD3021 is 400 mg once daily. What is the appropriate dose of Drug HD3021 for a 10-year-old male child that is 53 inches tall and weighs 78 pounds? Use Clark's Rule.

2. The adult dose of a drug is 150 mg twice daily for three days. How many milligrams (for a three-day course of therapy) should be dispensed to an 8-year-old female child that is 45 inches tall and weighs 57 pounds? Use Young's Rule.

3. Based on an adult dose of 600 mg, what is the appropriate dose for a 6-year-old boy that is 3 feet 4 inches tall and weighs 44 pounds? Use BSA Dosing.

4. If the adult dose of a drug is 1 gram, what is the appropriate dose for an 11-year-old child that weighs 100 pounds? Use Clark's Rule.

5. If the adult dose of a drug is 1 gram, what is the appropriate dose for an 11-year-old child that weighs 100 pounds? Use Young's Rule.

Practice Problem Answers

1. 208 mg
2. 360 mg (60 mg per dose x 6 doses)
3. 260 mg
4. 667 mg
5. 478 mg

CALCULATING IV DRIP RATES

To determine the drip rate for an intravenous (IV) infusion, you must first identify the volume (in milliliters) that must be infused into the patient and the length of time over which the infusion will take place. Once you know this information, all you need to do is convert the volume from milliliters to drops based on how many drops per milliliter the administration set delivers (e.g. a microdrip administration set delivers 60 drops/mL). Then you will have your answer. It is simple unit conversion – take the given information and convert the units until you get the drip rate (drops/minute).

TEST YOUR KNOWLEDGE

How many drops are there in one milliliter?

Typically, there are 15-20 drops per milliliter, but droppers or infusion administration sets can be specially manufactured to deliver anywhere from 10 to 60 drops per milliliter.

What is the name for an IV administration set that delivers 60 drops/mL?

Microdrip administration set.

EXAMPLE PROBLEMS

A 500 mL solution contains 2 grams of Drug X. How many mL/minute should be administered for the patient to receive 200 mg/hour?

Step 1: Determine the concentration of the infusion solution.

$$\frac{2 \text{ grams}}{500 \text{ mL}} \times \frac{1{,}000 \text{ mg}}{\text{gram}} = 4 \text{ mg/mL}$$

Step 2: Calculate the infusion rate in units of mL/min.

$$\frac{200 \text{ mg}}{\text{hr}} \times \frac{\text{mL}}{4 \text{ mg}} \times \frac{\text{hr}}{60 \text{ min}} = 0.83 \text{ mL/min}$$

Answer: 0.83 mL/min

In the problem above, what would the drip rate be if a drip set that delivers 60 drops/mL is utilized?

Solution:

$$\frac{0.83 \text{ mL}}{\text{min}} \times \frac{60 \text{ drops}}{\text{mL}} = 50 \text{ drops/min}$$

Answer: 50 drops/min

A patient is receiving 15,000 units of heparin per hour from an IV bag containing 250 mL of 100 unit/mL heparin. If the administration set delivers 20 drops/mL, how many drops is the patient receiving each minute?

Solution:

$$\frac{15{,}000\ \text{units}}{\text{hr}} \times \frac{\text{mL}}{100\ \text{units}} \times \frac{20\ \text{drops}}{\text{mL}} \times \frac{\text{hr}}{60\ \text{min}} = 50\ \text{drops/min}$$

Answer: 50 drops/min

Milrinone is dosed at 0.33 mcg/kg/min for a 210-pound patient. The infusion bag contains Milrinone 40 mg in 200 mL of D5W. What is the drip rate if the nurse uses a microdrip administration set (60 drops/mL)?

Solution:

$$\frac{0.33\ \text{mcg}}{\text{kg} \times \text{min}} \times \frac{210\ \text{lb}}{1} \times \frac{\text{kg}}{2.2\ \text{lb}} \times \frac{200\ \text{mL}}{40\ \text{mg}} \times \frac{1\ \text{mg}}{1{,}000\ \text{mcg}} \times \frac{60\ \text{drops}}{\text{mL}} = 9\ \text{drops/min}$$

Answer: 9 drops/min

A physician orders Vasopressin 30 milliunits/min. You dispense a 250-mL sterile admixture containing 25 units of Vasopressin in normal saline. If the administration set delivers 20 drops per milliliter, what is the appropriate drip rate?

Solution:

$$\frac{30\ \text{milliunits}}{\text{min}} \times \frac{250\ \text{mL}}{25\ \text{units}} \times \frac{\text{unit}}{1{,}000\ \text{milliunits}} \times \frac{20\ \text{drops}}{\text{mL}} = 6\ \text{drops/min}$$

Answer: 6 drops/min

PRACTICE PROBLEMS

1. What is the drip rate for a 250-mL bag of Vancomycin 1g in NSS if it is infused over one hour using a microdrip administration set (60 drops/milliliter)?

2. An administration set delivering 30 drops/mL was used to infuse a 160-mL bag of magnesium sulfate solution over the course of 120 minutes. What was the drip rate in units of drops/minute?

3. Drug M is available as a 100 mcg/1 mL infusion. If the patient weighs 176 pounds and Drug M is dosed at 10 mcg/kg/hr, what should the drip rate be if a microdrip administration set is used?

4. A patient receives 1 liter of Drug P over 24 hours. What is the drip rate if an administration set that delivers 19 drops/mL is used?

PRACTICE PROBLEM ANSWERS

1. 250 drops/minute
2. 40 drops/minute
3. 8 drops/minute
4. 13 drops/minute

CALCULATING DRUG PRICES

Calculating drug prices is a simple process of obtaining information and entering that information into an equation. To understand the drug pricing equation, you must first understand the terms and processes by which pharmacies purchase drug products.

DRUG PURCHASING PROCESS

1. Brand and Generic Manufacturers Sell Drug Products to Wholesale Distributors*
2. Wholesale Distributors Sell Drug Products to Pharmacies
3. Pharmacies Sell Drug Products to Customers

*There are many wholesale distributors, but the largest and most well-known among them include McKesson Corporation, Cardinal Health, and AmerisourceBergen. In some cases, the pharmacy may purchase certain drug products directly from the manufacturer. See "The Role of Wholesale Distributors" on the next page for more information.

DRUG PRICING TERMS

Average Wholesale Price (AWP)
The average price paid by a pharmacy to acquire a drug product from a wholesale distributor. Private and government insurance programs usually use AWP to calculate reimbursement rates for pharmacies.

Dispensing Fee
An amount added to the cost of each prescription dispensed by the pharmacy to cover direct and indirect costs associated with filling the prescription (e.g. employee wages, rent and utilities). The typical dispensing fee is roughly $2 - $12 per prescription.

Markup
An amount added to the cost of a drug for resale. A markup allows the pharmacy to profit from drug sales. Most businesses mathematically define the markup as a percentage of the acquisition cost. For instance, a 20% markup means the pharmacy will make a gross profit equal to 20% of the acquisition cost of the drug.

Retail Cost
Retail Cost is the total cost of the product charged to the customer. This price does not take into account a patient's prescription drug insurance and/or any discount cards or coupons they may use.

Wholesale Acquisition Cost (WAC)
The list price for a drug purchased from a manufacturer by a wholesale distributor or pharmacy. Since WAC reflects the list price, WAC does not take into account any discounts or rebates that purchasers are often able to obtain.

THE ROLE OF WHOLESALE DISTRIBUTORS

You may wonder why a wholesale distributor is necessary. Why not cut out the middleman? Hundreds of drug companies manufacture thousands of products all over the globe. It would be virtually impossible for a small business, such as an independent pharmacy, to organize and manage the ordering of drug products without the help of an intermediary (a wholesale distributor); however, for the most part, large retail chains *are* able to avoid the extra expense of a wholesale distributor. They do this by setting up their own distribution system in which they fulfill drug orders using company-owned warehouses and trucks. You will hear these referred to as "warehouse orders." However, they still tend to rely on wholesale distributors for rare items, lower cost brand name products, and/or next-day delivery.

WHERE TO OBTAIN DRUG PRICING INFORMATION

Several private companies publish up-to-date drug pricing information, but the largest and most well-known sources are:

- First DataBank
- Medi-Span
- Red Book*
- Gold Standard Drug Database

*Red Book is not to be confused with the Orange Book. The Red Book contains drug pricing information published by a private company, whereas the Orange Book is a therapeutic equivalence reference published by the federal government.

PRESCRIPTION DRUG PRICING EQUATION:

Retail Cost = [AWP x (1 + Markup*)] + Dispensing Fee
*Markup expressed as a decimal

Note: There are many intricacies and complexities to drug pricing terminology. Average Wholesale Price (AWP) is a commonly used term for the drug pricing equation, but the acquisition cost can be expressed using different terms. For instance, Actual Acquisition Cost (AAC) or Wholesale Acquisition Cost (WAC). All of these terms express acquisition cost in their own way and can serve as a reasonable substitute for AWP if a value for AWP is not given.

OVER-THE-COUNTER DRUG PRICING EQUATION

Retail Cost = AWP x (1 + Markup*)
*Markup expressed as a decimal

Note: The dispensing fee does not apply to OTC drugs.

EXAMPLE PROBLEMS

What is the Retail Cost (cost to the customer) of Drug X if AWP is $49.55, the Markup is 20%, and the Dispensing Fee is $10?

Retail Cost = [AWP x (1 + Markup)] + Dispensing Fee
Retail Cost = [$49.55 x (1 + 0.2)] + $10 = $69.46

Note: If Drug X were available OTC, there would not be a dispensing fee.

What is the AWP for Drug Y if the Retail Cost is $9.00, the Dispensing Fee is $2.00, and the Markup is 25%?

Retail Cost = [AWP x (1 + Markup)] + Dispensing Fee
AWP = (Retail Cost – Dispensing Fee) / (1 + Markup)
AWP = ($9.00 – $2.00) / (1 + 0.25) = $7 / 1.25 = $5.60

Note: To solve this problem, we had to rearrange the equation to solve for AWP.

What is the Retail Cost for 30 tablets of Citalopram if the Wholesale Acquisition Cost is $6.30 for 90 tablets and the Markup on this product is 50% with a $2 Dispensing Fee?

The WAC is for 90 tablets, but our patient is only getting 30. Before entering the information into the equation, we must reduce the WAC to reflect this difference. To accomplish this, we set up a proportion because the cost of 30 tablets will be proportional to the cost of 90 tablets. In our equation, variable "Y" represents the unknown cost of 30 tablets.

$$\frac{Y}{30 \text{ tablets}} = \frac{\$6.30}{90 \text{ tablets}}$$

Then cross multiply, and we get...

$$Y \times 90 \text{ tablets} = \$6.30 \times 30 \text{ tablets}$$

Then isolate Y by dividing each side by 90 tablets...

$$Y = \frac{\$6.30 \times 30 \text{ tablets}}{90 \text{ tablets}} = \$2.10$$

Retail Cost = [WAC x (1 + Markup)] + Dispensing Fee
Retail Cost = [$2.10 x (1 + 0.50)] + $2 = $5.15

Note: In this problem, AWP is unknown; however, as we noted beneath the "Prescription Drug Pricing Equation" on the previous page, WAC is a suitable substitute for AWP when AWP is not available.

What is the OTC Retail Cost for a bottle of 100 caplets of acetaminophen 500 mg if the Average Wholesale Price is $2.25 and the Markup is 200%?

Retail Cost = AWP x (1 + Markup)
Retail Cost = $2.25 x (1 + 2.00) = $6.75

Note: Make sure you use the "Over-The-Counter Drug Pricing Equation" for this one, and remember that only products dispensed from the pharmacy include a dispensing fee.

PRACTICE PROBLEMS

1. What is the Retail Cost of Drug B if the AWP is $20, the Dispensing Fee is $8, and the Markup is 50%?

2. What is the WAC of Drug C if the Retail Cost is $99.96, the Markup is 15%, and the Dispensing Fee is $7.50?

3. The pharmacy you work for dispenses a 30-tablet bottle of ibuprofen 800 mg for their favorite customer, Bob. The AWP is $5, the Markup is 100%, and the Dispensing Fee is $5. Bob wants to pay one-half of the Retail Cost with cash and the other half with a credit card. How much cash will Bob need?

4. What is the Retail Cost of a twin pack of OTC Robitussin if the AWP for the twin pack is $3 and the Markup is 400%?

PRACTICE PROBLEM ANSWERS

1. $38
2. $80.40
3. $7.50
4. $15

REPACKAGING MEDICATIONS

Many regulations address drug packaging and labeling (e.g. FDA Compliance Policy Guideline CPG Sec 430-100). From a regulatory point of view, the easiest thing to do is leave medications in the stock bottle (as supplied by the manufacturer) until the time of dispensing; however, there are undeniable benefits to repackaging. These benefits mainly apply to hospitals and other inpatient facilities. By transferring medications to unit-dose (single dose) packages, each dose obtains its own identifying label, helping inpatient facilities ensure the right drug is going to the right patient. Additionally, unit-dose packaging protects individual doses from the moisture and contamination. Consequently, the pharmacy can retrieve and re-dispense unused doses, thereby reducing waste.

For the reasons described above, it is common for pharmacies, particularly in a hospital setting, to repackage medications. The process of repackaging is simple and merely involves transferring individual doses (e.g. one tablet or capsule, or one or two teaspoons of a liquid) from a medication stock bottle into smaller, single use packages. Once the pharmacy transfers a medication from its original stock bottle into unit-dose packages, the stability of the drug falls into question. Will the drug be stable in this new environment? The repackaging material may accelerate the expiration of the drug. Pharmacies can perform stability tests, but these tests can be expensive and, in most cases, impractical. As an alternative, the FDA suggests assigning a beyond-use date (BUD) equal to six (6) months, provided this does not exceed 25% of the time remaining between the date of repackaging and the manufacturer-assigned expiration date printed on the label of the stock bottle.

Pharmacies can only use the 6-month beyond-use date shortcut for non-sterile liquid and solid dosage forms. In addition, the product must come from a previously unopened stock bottle, and the entire contents of the stock bottle must be repackaged in one operation. The repackaging process and subsequent storage of the product must comply with the manufacturer specifications for storage and handling (typically room temperature with relative humidity 75% or less). This information can be located in the package insert of any given drug. Pharmacy technicians can only repackage medications under the direct supervision of a licensed pharmacist, and most states require maintenance of a repackaging log that documents the details of repackaging (e.g. date repackaged, name of person repackaging). Take note that the FDA prohibits the repackaging of nitroglycerin sublingual tablets and other products with known stability issues.

SUMMARY OF UNIT-DOSE PACKAGE LABEL REQUIREMENTS

- Drug name & strength
- Beyond-use date
- Lot number
- Name and location of repackager
- Statement indicating special dosage form characteristics, if applicable (e.g. chewable, extended-release)
- NDC number (recommended, not required)
- If greater than one, the number of unit doses contained in each package
- For controlled substances, the statement "warning: may be habit forming" along with the controlled substance symbol (e.g. C-II, C-III, C-IV, or C-V)
- For prescription drugs, "Rx Only" or a similar statement

STERILE COMPOUNDING

In the process of treating medical problems, we need to be careful not to expose patients to disease-causing microorganisms. For drugs administered by way of the gastrointestinal tract, like oral capsules and tablets, development of a strictly sterile drug product is not necessary because acid in the stomach kills most bacteria. Additionally, the intestinal wall acts as a barrier to prevent ingested bacteria from entering the bloodstream. In essence, the stomach and intestines work like a filter. For drug infusions, sterility is very important since impurities are not filtered out by the stomach and intestines. If there are disease-causing microorganisms in an intravenous (IV) infusion, they will enter the bloodstream directly, and then use the circulating blood as a means of transportation to spread throughout the body, causing infection and disease.

What does the tem "aseptic" mean?
Without organisms (i.e. sterile).

What is a beyond use date (BUD)?
A beyond-use date is the date after which a compounded medication should not be used. Beyond-use dates are typically short (i.e. days, weeks, or months) compared to expiration dates which are usually one or more years. See page 224 for more details.

True or false. A beyond use date and an expiration date are the same thing.
False. Manufacturers assign expiration dates to manufactured products, whereas beyond use dates are assigned to compounded and repackaged drug products.

What is the technical term for a pharmacy clean room?
The buffer area.

What chapter of the United States Pharmacopoeia (USP) provides guidance on preparing compounded sterile products?
USP Chapter 797 (not to be confused with USP Chapter 795, which covers non-sterile compounding).

What is the purpose of USP Chapter 797?
To prevent patients from receiving contaminated infusions.

Personal Protective Equipment (PPE)
When compounding sterile products, it is important to follow USP Chapter 797 guidelines to assure the quality of the final product and prevent contamination by bacteria, fungi, viruses, particulate matter, etc. Next to thorough handwashing, one of the most important steps a pharmacy technician can take to reduce the likelihood of contaminating sterile products is to wear the appropriate personal protective equipment (PPE or "garb") at all times when in the clean room.
Appropriate PPE includes:

- Gown
- Shoe Covers
- Face Mask
- Beard Cover (if applicable)
- Hair Cover
- Gloves

What does it mean to "don" something?
To "don" means to put something on (e.g. to put on an article of clothing).

What is the proper order of donning PPE (also known as "garbing")?
1. Shoe Covers
2. Hair Cover
3. Beard Cover (if applicable)
4. Face Mask
****Handwashing****
5. Gown
6. Gloves

Note: In general, you want to put on your clean room garb in the order of dirtiest to cleanest (shoes are assumed to be the dirtiest and washed hands are considered to be the cleanest).

When should PPE be removed?
Only after exiting the clean room.

What is the most common cause of contamination?
Touch contamination (i.e. contact with the hand contaminates the sterile product).

When washing your hands prior to preparing a compounded sterile product (CSP), what should you use?

A. Antibacterial soap and scalding hot water.
B. Antibacterial soap and warm water.
C. Antibacterial soap and cold water.

Answer:
B. Antibacterial soap and warm water.

What is the proper procedure for hand washing prior to entering the clean room?
Wash the hands and arms all the way up to the elbows vigorously for at least 30 seconds paying special attention to the fingernails and the spaces between the fingers.

According to USP Chapter 797, what items are prohibited in the buffer area?

- Makeup
- Jewelry
- Watches
- Nail polish
- Artificial nails

Does USP Chapter 797 permit eating or drinking in the buffer area?
No.

ISO CLASSIFICATION

The International Organization for Standardization (ISO) defines air qualities based on the number of particles in the air. There are three classes of air quality relevant to pharmacy. The names and definitions are as follows:

ISO class 8 – 3,520,000 particles or less (of size 0.5 microns or larger) per cubic meter of air.
ISO class 7 – 352,000 particles or less (of size 0.5 microns or larger) per cubic meter of air.
ISO class 5 – 3,520 particles or less (of size 0.5 microns or larger) per cubic meter of air.

Note: The exact definitions are not important. Just be aware that lower ISO classifications indicate fewer particles and cleaner air.

WHY ALL THE PRECAUTIONS?

When compounding sterile products for infusion, it is important to prevent particles from entering the preparation. When particles or contaminants are infused into a patient's bloodstream, they can clog up a blood vessel or cause an infection. The last thing we want to do is introduce a loose hair, piece of glass, or virus into a sick patient's vein. This is precisely why we use clean rooms and laminar airflow hoods. These tools create an environment with ultra-low particle air ideal for preparing sterile, particle-free infusion products.

ISO CLASSIFICATION BASED ON LOCATION

LOCATION	AIR QUALITY
Ante Area / Ante Room	ISO Class 8
Buffer Area / Clean Room	ISO Class 7
Laminar Airflow Hood (LAFH)	ISO Class 5

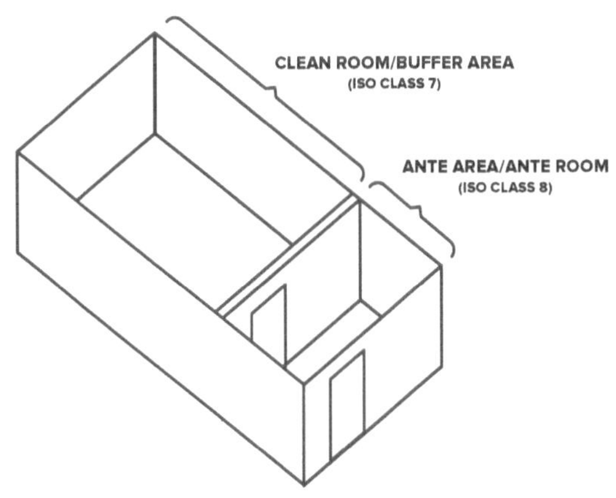

There are 5 levels of risk associated with compounded sterile products. What are the risk levels and how are they defined?

1. Immediate-use category
- Prepared using aseptic technique, but not in a clean room.
- Takes less than 1 hour to compound the formulation.
- Can be administered within 1 hour of compounding.
- Only for emergency situations where low-risk compounding procedures would lead to an unreasonable delay in therapy.
  - BUD 1 hour (refrigeration or room temperature)

2. Low-risk level
- Prepared using aseptic technique in a clean room.*
- Simple admixtures (up to 3 ingredients added with 2 entries into the infusion bag) using closed system transfer methods.
- Ingredients are sterile.
  - BUD 48 hours (room temperature)
  - BUD 14 days (refrigeration)
  - BUD 45 days (frozen at a temperature ≤ 10°C)

3. Low-risk level with < 12 hour BUD
- Prepared in an ISO Class 5 LAFH, but not in a clean room.
- Simple admixtures (up to 3 ingredients added with 2 entries into the infusion bag) using closed system transfer methods.
- Ingredients are sterile.
- Must be administered within 12 hours of preparation.
  - BUD 12 hours (refrigeration or room temperature)

4. Medium-risk level
- Prepared using aseptic technique in a clean room.
- Complex manipulations (several ingredients and entries into the bag) or extensive amount of time required to compound (e.g. TPNs and batch compounded preparations).
- Formulations that are used over several days.
- Ingredients are sterile.
  - BUD 30 hours (room temperature)
  - BUD 9 days (refrigeration)
  - BUD 45 days (frozen at a temperature ≤ 10°C)

5. High-risk level
- Prepared in a clean room.
- Ingredients are not sterile (e.g. bulk powders), or compounding method involves open system transfers.
- Improper garb.
  - BUD 24 hours (room temperature)
  - BUD 3 days (refrigeration)
  - BUD 45 days (frozen at a temperature ≤ 10°C)

*Clean rooms (buffer areas) provide ISO Class 7 air quality and contain ISO Class 5 laminar airflow hoods (LAFHs), and they are located directly adjacent to an ISO Class 8 ante area.

The principles of sterile compounding are referred to as ____________.
Aseptic technique.

Highlights of aseptic technique:

⇒ Allow the laminar airflow hood (LAFH) to run for 30 minutes before compounding if not in continuous use.

⇒ Clean the LAFH with 70% isopropyl alcohol (wipe from top to bottom and back to front; clean all surfaces inside the hood except the screen housing the HEPA filter).

⇒ Remove items from their packaging *before* placing them inside the hood.

⇒ Perform sterile manipulations at least 6 inches inside the outer edge of the hood (see the LAFH illustration below).

⇒ Do not place any objects between the HEPA filter and work area.

⇒ Swab surfaces with 70% isopropyl alcohol prior to puncturing (e.g. the rubber stopper on a vial; see illustration at top of next page).

⇒ Do not block or disrupt the flow of air over the critical sites with your hands/fingers when manipulating the objects inside the hood (see illustration at bottom of next page – notice how hand/finger positioning does not block the airflow from the LAFH).

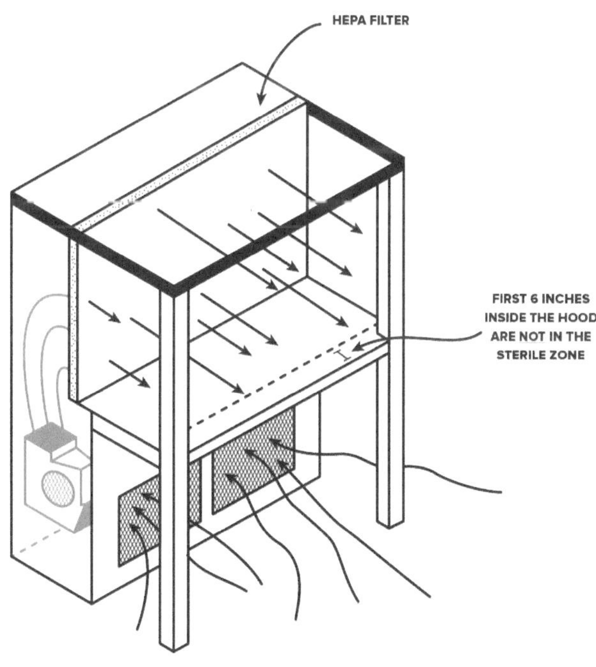

LAMINAR AIRFLOW HOOD (LAFH)

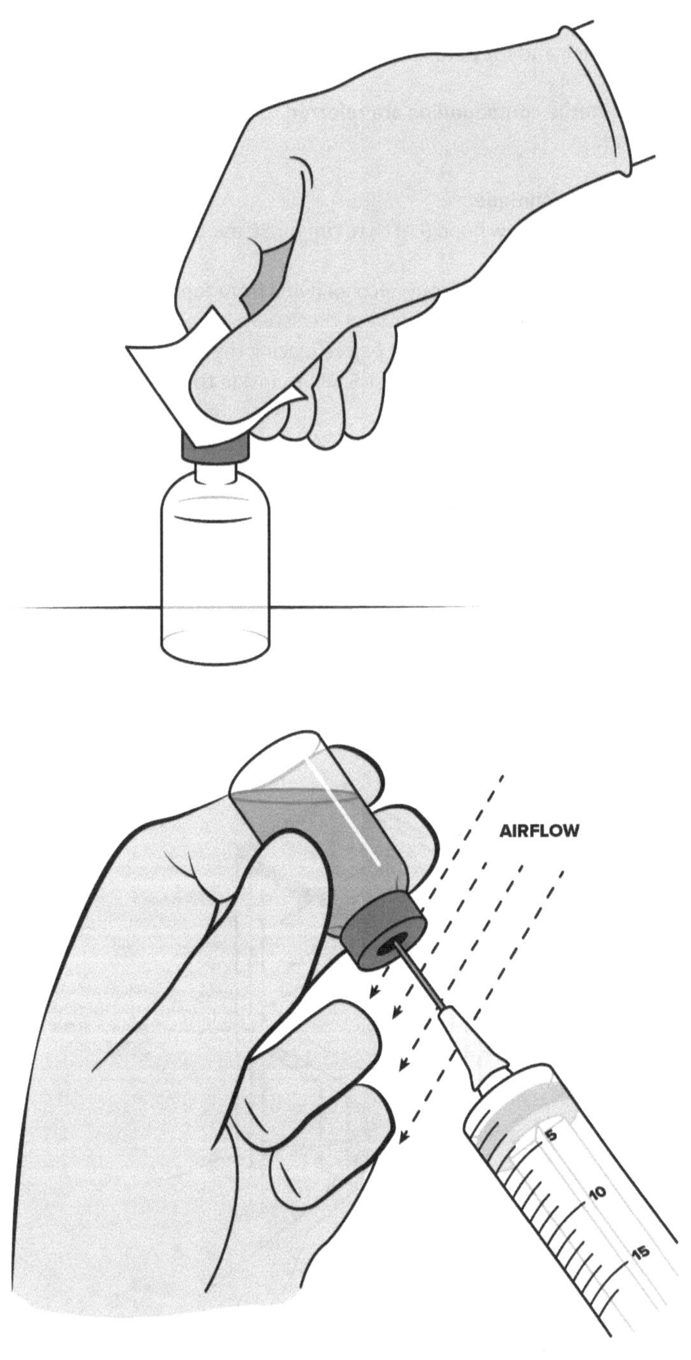
AIRFLOW
5
10
15

What is the "critical site?"
The critical site is an opening that provides a pathway between the contents of a sterile product container and the environment. A common example of this is the rubber stopper on a vial and the needle of a syringe used to obtain the contents from the vial. When the needle punctures the rubber stopper, it creates an opening between the sterile contents of the vial and the surrounding environment.

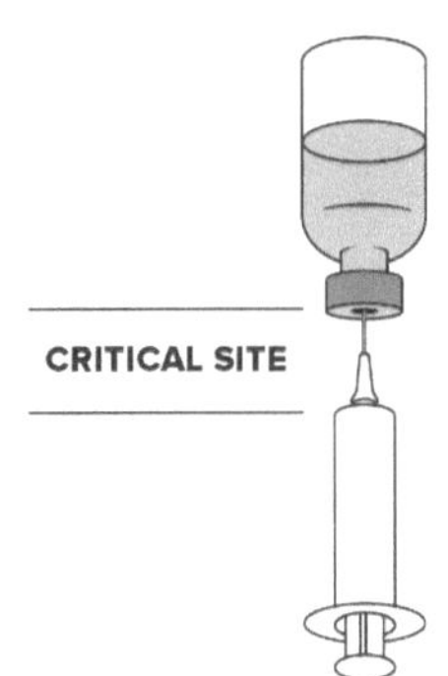

Sterile alcohol swabs are soaked in what type of alcohol?
70% isopropyl alcohol.

What type of container must be used for the disposal of needles?
A red sharps container.

What is the purpose of a laminar airflow hood (LAFH)?
To create an environment with a very low concentration of particles and microorganisms so formulations safe enough for human infusion can be prepared.
Note: LAFH can also be abbreviated as LAFW (laminar airflow workbench).

How many air filters is a LAFH equipped with?
2 air filters (1 regular filter and 1 HEPA filter).

What is a HEPA filter?
HEPA stands for "High Efficiency Particulate Air." HEPA filters remove 99.97% of particles from the air that are 0.3 microns (micrometers) or larger.

How frequently should you wipe or spray a HEPA filter with alcohol?
Never. This would damage the filter membrane.

The LAFH must be turned on and left running for how many minutes prior to use?
30 minutes.

Besides being running it for 30 minutes, what else must be done prior to using a LAFH?
It must be cleaned with 70% isopropyl alcohol.

How frequently should a LAFH be cleaned with alcohol when in constant use?
Every 30 minutes.

To assure that filtered air reaches the critical site, you must work at least __ inches inside the LAFH.
6.

In a LAFH, you want to avoid placing your hands or other objects behind the materials you are working with to prevent ________________.
Airflow obstruction.

What type of hood should be used for compounding chemotherapy infusions?
A biological safety cabinet.

Infusion filters are available with many different pore sizes. Smaller pore sizes filter out more unwanted particles, but are more prone to clogging. What are some examples of unwanted particles that filters are helpful in removing?
Glass particles, rubber fragments, dust, clothing fibers, fungi, and bacteria.

What is a micron?
A micron is a measure of length equal to one one-millionth of one meter.

What pore size is optimal for removing microorganisms, such as bacteria and fungi?
0.22 μm (referred to as a "0.22 micron filter").

What is total parenteral nutrition (TPN)?
A sterile formulation of liquid nutrients delivered by intravenous infusion.

What is the difference between total parenteral nutrition (TPN) and total nutrient admixture (TNA)?
TPNs are a 2-in-1 mixture of amino acids and dextrose (plus electrolytes), whereas TNAs are a 3-in-1 mixture which includes the above plus a fat (lipid) component.

Note: We commonly hear people referring to TNAs and TPNs as though they are synonymous, even though *technically* they are not the same.

What would happen if you used a 0.22 micron filter on a TNA (3-in-1)?
The filter would be clogged by the lipid component of the TNA.

What is the optimal pore size for filtering an infusion that contains lipids (as found in a TNA infusion)?
1.2 microns (1.2 μm).

What are the benefits and drawbacks of a 1.2 micron filter?
BENEFITS:
- Good flow of emulsified fat and other contents through the filter.
- Low probability of clogging.
- Fungi are filtered out.

DRAWBACK:
- Bacteria and other materials smaller than 1.2 microns are not filtered out.

What is the most important compatibility consideration in TNA preparation?
The incompatibility between calcium and phosphate. If the concentration of these two ions is too high, insoluble precipitates will form. Due to the lipid content, TNAs are white and opaque, making it nearly impossible to see calcium phosphate precipitates.

How can you minimize the risk of calcium phosphate precipitation?
By adding phosphate early in the compounding process and adding calcium last.

What issue must be considered when including insulin in a TPN or TNA?
Up to 50% of the insulin will bind to the surface of the inside of the bag and administration set (tubing).

What can happen when vitamin C (ascorbic acid) is included in a TPN or TNA?
Over time, ascorbic acid degrades to oxalate, which quickly binds with calcium to form an insoluble precipitate called calcium oxalate.

Why are we concerned about precipitate formation?
Precipitates are solid particles. If a solid particle is infused into a patient's bloodstream, it can get stuck in a blood vessel and block the flow of blood. This can lead to a cardiovascular event (e.g. heart attack, stroke, pulmonary embolism).

Many vials say "single-dose" on the label, indicating that the contents are preservative-free. Once the stopper of a single-dose vial is punctured, in what time frame must you to use the contents of the vial?

- If the vial is stored in less than ISO Class 5 air, you have 1 hour to use it.
- If stored in ISO Class 5 or cleaner air, you have 6 hours to use it.

ANATOMY OF A SYRINGE & NEEDLE

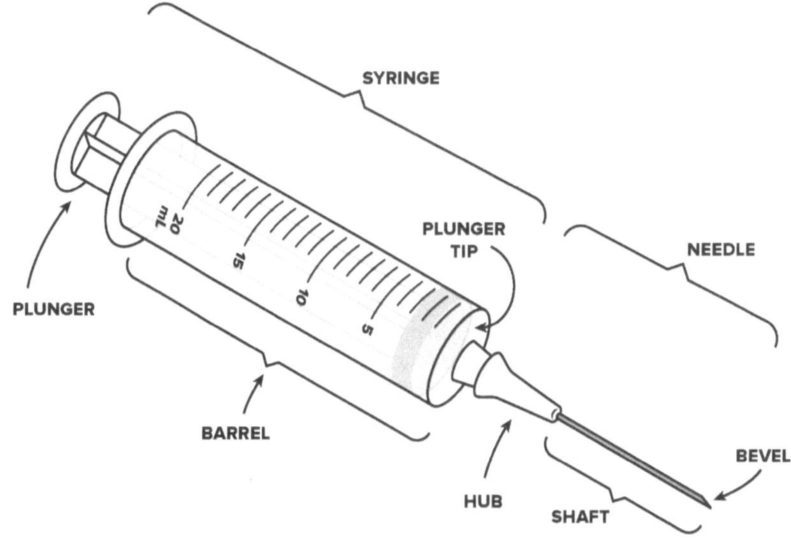

UNDERSTANDING NEEDLE GAUGES

30 Gauge Needle 16 Gauge Needle

Key point: Gauge size is inversely proportional to the diameter of the needle lumen. In other words... the higher the gauge, the thinner the needle.

SELECTING THE RIGHT SYRINGE FOR THE JOB

The syringes we use for sterile admixture are available in many sizes, including 1, 3, 5, 10, 20, 30, and 60 milliliters. When measuring any volume of liquid, we generally want to use the smallest syringe that can hold the desired volume; however, it is important to remember that syringes can be used accurately to measure up to one-half of the smallest marked unit. For instance, if you were using a 10-mL syringe with 10 hash marks, where each hash mark represented 1 milliliter, then that syringe could be used to measure accurately up to the nearest half (0.5) milliliter.

Given what we now know, would we be able to use the syringe pictured below to measure a volume of 11 milliliters? Why or why not?

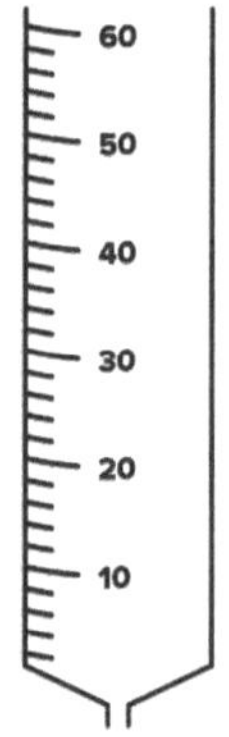

Yes. Syringes can measure accurately up to one-half of the smallest marked unit, and since the syringe pictured above displays a marking for each 2-mL increment, it can accurately measure to the nearest 1 mL. Even though this 60-mL syringe would do the job, we would *prefer* to use a 20-mL syringe. Remember, our options are 1, 3, 5, 10, 20, 30, and 60 milliliters. A 20-mL syringe would be the smallest syringe that could hold 11 milliliters.

SIGNS OF INCOMPATIBILITY

When mixing medications for IV administration, it is important to look for signs of incompatibility. What are some common signs of incompatibility?

- Gas formation (bubbles)
- Precipitate formation (solid particles)
- Turbidity (cloudiness)
- Color change

PATIENT-CONTROLLED ANALGESIA (PCA)

When a patient is in severe pain, such as in the days following major surgery, our goal is to treat their pain as quickly and effectively as possible. The most effective pain medications are opioid analgesics (e.g. morphine, hydromorphone, and fentanyl). While very effective, high doses of an opioid can induce sedation and suppress breathing. Furthermore, they are controlled substances, which means they have potential for abuse and addiction. Patient-controlled analgesia (PCA) places pain management in the hands of the patient. When the patient is in pain, he/she presses a button that triggers an electronic infusion pump to administer an intravenous (IV) injection. For example, if a patient received a prescription for a fentanyl PCA pump at the dose of 10 mcg up to every 8 minutes, then the patient would be able to press a button and receive 10 mcg of fentanyl through an IV line up to every 8 minutes. The pump would not administer the dose unless a full 8 minutes elapsed from the time of the previous dose. This 8-minute time period is called the "lockout interval." The lockout interval makes it possible for the patient to receive pain medication on-demand, while minimizing the risk of abuse, addiction, and side effects.

BEYOND-USE DATES

Beyond-use dates (BUDs) are important for non-sterile repackaged drug products, compounded preparations, and opened vials containing sterile medication for injection. We already discussed BUDs for repackaged medications (see page 212), so this section will focus on BUDs for compounded preparations and vials containing sterile medication for injection. First, we will discuss the importance of the BUD for compounded preparations.

Each ingredient in a compounded preparation has a manufacturer-assigned expiration date, but the final compounded product has characteristics that are often very different from the characteristics of any individual ingredient. For instance, the viscosity, the water content, the concentration of preservatives will all be different. Additionally, the container used to store the final compounded product is inevitably different from the individual ingredient storage containers. Over time, chemical reactions can occur between these various components, ultimately affecting the strength, quality, purity, and stability of the final compounded product. For that reason, it is necessary to determine a reasonable time through which we can be confident that the final compounded product will maintain the expected level of strength, quality, purity and stability – the beyond-use date.

Now, we will address beyond-use dates for opened vials containing sterile medication for injection. As with any other medication, a manufacturer assigns an expiration date for each container of medication and communicates this information to the pharmacy by stamping the expiration date on the container label. This expiration date is the manufacturer's guarantee that the contents of the container will be sterile, effective, and otherwise safe until the expiration date... provided the pharmacy stores the medication according to the conditions specified on the label. The instant a needle enters the vial the expiration date no longer applies. Aseptic technique is required for sterile compounding and admixture manipulations, but, regardless of how well the compounder adheres to the principles of aseptic technique, a certain amount of bacteria will inevitably enter the vial and begin to reproduce. The only question is... should we deem the contents of the vial to be "contaminated" or otherwise unusable?

Unless the vial says "multi-dose" on the label, assume the vial is single-use only. For single-use vials, we must discard any remaining content soon after initial use. The reason being, single-use vials do not contain preservatives to protect the contents from bacterial proliferation... and, as previously mentioned, some bacteria will infiltrate an open vial and multiply, even if the compounder uses proper aseptic technique. Multi-dose vials do contain preservatives. For that reason, disposal of unused portions of medication is not necessary... as long as aseptic technique is used; however, preservatives have their limitations. Unless specified otherwise in the labeling, multi-dose vials have a BUD of 28 days after initial use. As covered elsewhere in this study guide, this same BUD applies to most vials of insulin, which are indeed multi-dose vials.

PARENTERAL ADMINISTRATION ROUTES

Parenteral administration routes give us the ability to deliver a medication into the body by way other than the gastrointestinal tract (i.e. oral or rectal administration). Technically, a parenteral administration route would include anything other than oral or rectal administration (e.g. transdermal, ophthalmic, nasal, and injectable); however, in the pharmacy setting, parenteral generally means injectable. For that reason, this section will provide a review of injectable administration routes. For the first three administration routes listed below, we have included information regarding the appropriate needle size. The reason being, pharmacies often dispense needles and syringes for patients who self-administer injectable medications such as insulin and vitamin B12. Retail pharmacists also administer immunizations using subcutaneous, intramuscular, and intradermal injection techniques. As a pharmacy technician, you can better aid the pharmacist if you are familiar with the needle sizes used for the different injection routes, for instance when ordering replenishment supplies and helping patients purchase needs and syringes for self-administration of insulin.

Subcutaneous (SC or SQ)

Subcutaneous injections deliver medication into the tissue just underneath the skin where the medication is absorbed into the bloodstream and carried throughout the body where it exerts its effect. The optimal needle size for a subcutaneous injection is 25 – 30 gauge with a length of 1/4 inch to 5/8 inch. Obese patients may require a longer needle. The most common injection sites for subcutaneous injections include the thigh, abdomen, and outer upper arm. Insulin is an example of a medication administered by subcutaneous injection

Intramuscular (IM)

Intramuscular injections deliver medication deep below the skin into the muscle tissue where the medication is slowly absorbed into the bloodstream. The optimal needle size for an intramuscular injection is 19 to 25 gauge with a length of 1 inch to 1 & 1/2 inches. Obese patients may require a longer needle. The most common injection sites for intramuscular injections include the deltoid muscle (upper arm) and the gluteus maximus. Vitamin B12 (cyanocobalamin) injections are typically administered by intramuscular injection.

Intradermal (ID)

Intradermal injections deliver pharmaceutical products into the skin layers, just below the outer surface of the skin. Since the needle does not go deep, this type of injection does not cause much pain; however, only a small volume of liquid can be injected. Consequently, not many products are administered by intradermal injection. The most common needles size for an intradermal injection is 23 to 26 gauge with a short length of only 1/4 to 3/8 inch. One example of an intradermal injection is the Tuberculin Skin Test, a diagnostic test used to determine whether an individual has a tuberculosis infection.

Intravenous (IV)

Intravenous infusions are the most common type of sterile product prepared by pharmacies. Unlike the previous routes we discussed, IV infusions are administered directly into the bloodstream. In a hospital setting, many antibiotics, cardiac drugs, and rehydration fluids are given this way.

Epidural

Epidurals deliver medication into the area near the spinal cord. Epidural infusions are commonly used for labor pain during childbirth and for anesthesia during orthopedic surgery or C-sections. Directly exposing nerve tissue to medication preservatives will cause nerve damage in many cases. For that reason, the medications used in epidurals must be preservative-free (PF). The active ingredients in an epidural usually include an opioid analgesic (e.g. fentanyl or hydromorphone) and an anesthetic (e.g. bupivacaine).

Intrathecal (IT)

The difference between an epidural and an intrathecal infusion is that epidurals deliver medication to the space just near the spinal cord; whereas, intrathecal infusions deliver medication directly into the spinal fluid. Intrathecal infusions are used for the treatment of cancer. They are also used for delivering pain medication in a fashion similar to epidurals. As with epidurals, intrathecal infusions should only contain preservative-free ingredients.

Note: Other injectable routes of administration exist, such as intra-arterial, intra-cardiac, and intramedullary, but these routes are reserved for special situations that are too advanced for the context of the exam and this study guide.

SPECIAL PROCEDURES FOR HAZARDOUS DRUGS

What is a hazardous drug?
A hazardous drug is a medication that can cause harm to human or animal life. For example, exposure to a hazardous drug may cause reproductive toxicity, organ damage, birth defects, and/or cancer.

In which drug classes do we find most hazardous drugs?
Cancer chemotherapy, antivirals, immunosuppressants, hormones, and certain anticonvulsants.

Why would a patient receive a hazardous drug?
Consider a patient with cancer. The cancer, if left untreated, could grow and spread very quickly. Now imagine that there is a drug that could slow, and potentially stop, the cancer growth, but this drug is known to cause liver toxicity. For our patient with cancer, the benefit of slowing or stopping the cancer is likely to outweigh the risk of liver toxicity.

When handling hazardous drugs, healthcare workers should follow __________________ and any recommendations included in the manufacturer's ________________________.

- Standard precautions
- Material safety data sheet (MSDS)

What are the standard precautions that should be followed by healthcare workers when handling hazardous drugs?

- Store hazardous drugs in a well-ventilated area separate from all other inventory.
- Wear chemotherapy gloves whenever handling hazardous drugs (e.g. when receiving, stocking, counting, preparing for administration, and disposing).
- Perform sterile compounding activities with hazardous drugs in an ISO class 5 biological safety cabinet or compounding aseptic containment isolator.
    - **Note:** The safety cabinet or containment isolator used for compounding hazardous drugs must be physically separate from other sterile compounding preparation areas.
- Wear appropriate personal protective equipment (PPE) when compounding products that contain hazardous drugs.
    - Gown.
    - Face mask.
    - Eye protection.*
    - Hair cover.
    - Shoe covers.
    - Double-gloving with sterile chemotherapy gloves.*

*Precautions not routinely recommended for compounding non-hazardous sterile drug products.

Why is it necessary for healthcare workers to follow standard precautions when handling hazardous drugs?
When healthy individuals are exposed to a hazardous drug, they risk experiencing the potential adverse effects associated with using the drug, but with no therapeutic benefit.

What organizations provide information regarding the storage, handling, and disposal of hazardous drugs?

- United States Pharmacopoeia (USP)
- American Society of Health-System Pharmacists (ASHP)
- National Institute for Occupational Safety and Health (NIOSH)
- Occupational Safety and Health Administration (OSHA)

What information is provided in a product's material safety data sheet (MSDS)?

- Chemical and physical properties.
- Health, safety, fire, and environmental hazards.
- Information on what to do if the product is accidentally spilled.

Material Safety Data Sheets are for ____________________ & ____________________.

- Workers that will potentially be exposed to chemicals.
- Emergency response personnel (e.g. firefighters).

Who is responsible for making MSDSs available to employees?
The employer.

What type of container must be used for disposal of needles and syringes with hazardous drug residue?
Chemotherapy sharps container.

How does one distinguish a standard sharps container from a chemotherapy sharps container?
Standard sharps containers are red & chemotherapy sharps containers are yellow.

What is the purpose of a black pharmaceutical waste container?
Black pharmaceutical waste containers are used for the disposal of bulk hazardous drug waste (e.g. disposal of a partially empty vial of a cancer chemotherapy drug).

All areas where hazardous drugs are routinely handled must contain:

- Hazardous drug spill kits
- Containment bags
- Disposal containers

SUMMARY OF PHARMACEUTICAL WASTE CONTAINERS

	Red Container	Yellow Container	Black Container
Standard Sharps Waste	✓		
Sharps Waste with Hazardous Drug Residue		✓	
Bulk Hazardous Drug Waste			✓

What supplies should be included in a hazardous drug spill kit?

- Material to absorb about 1,000 mL of liquid
  - Plastic-backed, absorbent spill cleanup pads
  - Disposable towels
- Personal protective equipment (PPE)
  - Two (2) pairs of gloves
  - Gown
  - Shoe covers
  - Face shield
- Two (2) or more sealable plastic hazardous waste disposal bags
- One (1) disposable scooper and one (1) puncture-resistant container for collecting and disposing of broken glass.

Note: all spill cleanup materials must be disposed of as hazardous waste.

What steps should you take in the event of exposure to a hazardous drug by direct skin or eye contact?

- Call for help (if necessary).
- Remove any contaminated clothing.
- Wash affected eye(s) with water for at least 15 minutes.
- Clean affected skin with soap and water. Rinse well.
- Seek medical attention and document the exposure.

HAZARDOUS DRUGS – SELECT EXAMPLES

DRUG CLASS	GENERIC DRUG NAME
Cancer Chemotherapy	Anastrozole Bicalutimide Cisplatin Exemestane 5-Fluorouracil Letrozole Mercaptopurine Methotrexate Oxaliplatin Tamoxifen Vinblastine Vincristine
Antivirals	Abacavir Entecavir Ganciclovir Valganciclovir Zidovudine
Immune System Suppressants	Azathioprine Cyclosporine Mycophenolate Sirolimus Tacrolimus

PHARMACY TECHNICIAN CERTIFICATION

Renewal Requirements

Once you become a Certified Pharmacy Technician (CPhT) by passing the ExCPT exam, you must renew your certification every 2 years to keep it active. See below for a quick summary of the renewal requirements. More information regarding renewal is available at www.NHAnow.com.

- Obtain 20 hours of continuing education (CE) in the 2 years prior to recertification
  - Including at least 1 hour on the subject of pharmacy law
  - Keep CE participation certificates as evidence of completion*
- Submit the NHA ExCPT Recertification Application Form
  - Available at www.NHAnow.com
  - Include payment of $40 recertification fee

*The NHA may randomly select pharmacy technicians to audit their continuing education credits. For that reason, it is important to keep participation certificates as evidence that you have actually completed the required amount of continuing education.

CONGRATULATIONS!

Congratulations! You are almost prepared to take the ExCPT exam. Do not quit preparing until you feel confident. Be sure to memorize all you can. Only you can accurately judge your level of readiness. Once you are finished with this study guide, proceed to test your knowledge and skills with our full-length practice exam.

Tips to help you perform well on the actual exam:

- If you have never been to the testing center where your exam is scheduled, drive there a few days ahead of time so you know how to get there and what the parking situation is like.
- Ensure you are well-rested, well-hydrated, and well-fed on exam day.
- Do not rush through the exam; remain calm.
- The test is multiple-choice, so if you do not know the right answer to a question/problem, then eliminate some of the choices that you know are incorrect.
- When you don't know an answer and you are forced to guess, do not select an answer you have never heard of (e.g. if you have it narrowed down to: "A. Diabetes" or "B. Diffuse Intravascular Coagulation," then choose "A. Diabetes"). The answer is probably easier than you think.
- As previously mentioned, the entire exam is multiple-choice (including the math problems). Usually multiple-choice exams benefit the test-taker, but be careful! When math problems are presented in a multiple-choice format, the various choices are often designed to trick and deceive you. My advice for math problems is to solve them and double check your answer using a calculator before even looking at the answer options.
- Remember, you will get 130 minutes (2 hours and 10 minutes) to complete the exam and you will need to earn a scaled score of 390 to pass. That means you have to get about 70% of the questions correct. The practice exam on the following pages contains 120 problems, just like the actual ExCPT exam. For the purposes of this practice exam, assume each problem is worth one point. For answers that are completely or partially wrong, you do not receive the point. When you are finished, add up all of your points and divide that quantity by 120. You will get a decimal (something between 0.00 and 1.00). Multiply that number by 100%. For instance, if you answer 90 questions correct, divide 90 by 120, which equals 0.75. So take 0.75 and multiply that by 100%. That equals 75%, which would be an example of a passing score (> 70%).

Proceed with confidence!
-David Heckman, PharmD

STREAM ONLINE ExCPT EXAM PREP VIDEOS ON DEMAND

CPhT///ACADEMY

www.CPhTAcademy.com

PRACTICE EXAM

SET A TIMER FOR 2 HOURS AND 10 MINUTES

THEN PROCEED

1. Mr. Tucker weighs 65 kg. What is Mr. Tucker's weight in pounds?

A. 65 lb
B. 130 kg
C. 143 lb
D. 154 lb

2. If a bottle of Protonix® has a manufacturer-assigned expiration date of 09/2015, what is the last day it can be used?

A. August 31, 2015
B. September 1, 2015
C. September 30, 2015
D. October 1, 2015
E. None of the above

3. What is the generic drug name for Keppra®?

A. Lansoprazole
B. Lamotrigine
C. Ipratropium
D. Levetiracetam

4. Which task must be completed by a licensed pharmacist?

A. Accepting a new prescription from a patient.
B. Answering the telephone.
C. Counting tablets to fill a prescription for amlodipine.
D. Recommending an OTC medication for a patient.
E. All of the above.

5. Which class of FDA recall would be issued for a product that is unlikely to cause any adverse health effects?

A. Class I
B. Class II
C. Class III
D. Class IV

6. Which of the following tasks may be performed by a pharmacy technician?

A. Make a determination of therapeutic equivalency.
B. Evaluate the safety of drug therapy.
C. Administer an immunization.
D. Type a prescription label.

7. What is the primary role of the pharmacy technician?

A. Train pharmacy technician students.
B. Double-check the work of the pharmacist.
C. Assist the pharmacist.
D. Count pills.

8. Needles and syringes that have been used to compound a cancer chemotherapy infusion should be placed in which of the following waste containers...

A. Red sharps container
B. Yellow sharps container
C. Black pharmaceutical waste container
D. Waste basket

9. What is the purpose of rotating stock?

A. To ensure that patients are receiving the newest medication first.
B. To maintain a clean and orderly appearance in the pharmacy.
C. To decrease the emphasis on patient safety.
D. To ensure that drugs closer to expiration are dispensed first.

10. Which of the following agencies is responsible for enforcing the federal Controlled Substances Act (CSA)?

A. FDA
B. DEA
C. OSHA
D. FTC
E. None of the above

11. Which controlled substance schedule fits the following description?

Used medically; high potential for abuse and physical/psychological dependence.

A. Schedule I
B. Schedule II
C. Schedule III
D. Schedule IV
E. Schedule V

12. Look at prescription below. Is the prescriber's DEA number valid?

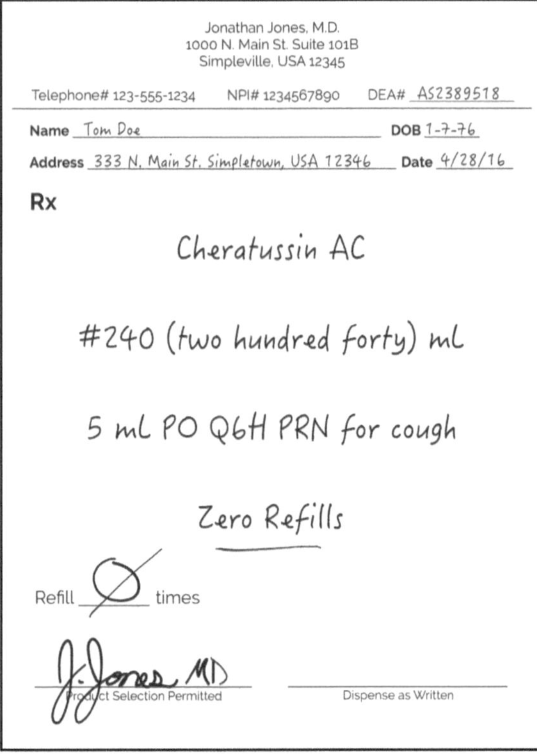
Jonathan Jones, M.D.
1000 N. Main St. Suite 101B
Simpleville, USA 12345

Telephone# 123-555-1234 NPI# 1234567890 DEA# AS2389518

Name Tom Doe DOB 1-7-76

Address 333 N. Main St. Simpletown, USA 12346 Date 4/28/16

Rx

Cheratussin AC

#240 (two hundred forty) mL

5 mL PO Q6H PRN for cough

Zero Refills

Refill Ø times

J. Jones, MD
Product Selection Permitted

Dispense as Written

A. Yes
B. No
C. Not enough information to answer the question

13. What is the maximum amount of pseudoephedrine one person may purchase in one day?

A. 2 grams
B. 3.6 grams
C. 7.5 grams
D. 9 grams
E. 5 boxes

14. What is the name of the form used to order Schedule II controlled substances?

A. DEA Form 41
B. DEA Form 222
C. Invoice
D. DEA Form 106
E. Pharmacy C-II Order Sheet

15. What is wrong with the prescription shown below?

James Smith, D.O.
Simplified Medical Clinic
10001 N. Main St. Suite 100A, Simple City, USA 24680
Telephone# 123-555-1234

Name Jane Doe Age 44

Address 555 South Main St. Anywhere, USA 10001 Date 3/30/16

Rx

Norco 5/325 mg tablets
60 (sixty)
Take i-ii PO Q4-6H PRN for pain

NR (1) 2 3 4 5 PRN

James Smith, D.O.

Prescriber must write "Brand Medically Necessary" on the prescription to prohibit generic substitution.

A. Refills cannot be issued for a Schedule II controlled substance.
B. The patient's state-issued ID number is not written on the prescription.
C. The prescriber's DEA number is not written on the prescription.
D. Both A & C.
E. All of the above.

16. What is the correct days' supply and DAW code to use when billing the patient's insurance for the prescription shown in question #15?

A. 15-day supply; DAW 9.
B. 10-day supply; DAW 1.
C. 8-day supply; DAW 0.
D. 5-day supply; DAW 0.
E. 7-day supply; DAW 0.

17. How many refills can be issued for a C-IV controlled substance prescription?

A. No refills.
B. Up to 5 refills.
C. Up to 6 refills.
D. Up to 12 refills.

18. Which of the following medications is not a Schedule III controlled substance?

A. AndroGel®
B. Suboxone®
C. Ambien®
D. Subutex®

19. Prescribers that issue buprenorphine (i.e. Suboxone® and Subutex®) prescriptions for treatment of narcotic drug addiction outside of a narcotics treatment facility must have a unique DEA number that begins with the __________.

A. Number 2
B. Letter X
C. Number 9
D. Letter Z

20. Which prescriber identification number is required for submitting insurance claims?

A. UPIN Number
B. NPI Number
C. DEA Number
D. Driver's License Number

21. What is the purpose of the Health Insurance Portability & Accountability Act (HIPAA)?

A. To require drug utilization reviews for Medicaid patients.
B. To protect children from serious injury caused by ingesting medications.
C. To prevent the use of pseudoephedrine in illegal drug production.
D. To protect the privacy of patient health information.

22. Which of the following practitioners would have limited prescribing authority (as opposed to full prescribing authority)?

A. Podiatrist
B. Nurse Practitioner
C. Dentist
D. Veterinarian

23. How did the Poison Prevention Packaging Act (PPPA) affect pharmacy practice?

A. It required prescription drug packaging to be made of red cellophane.
B. It placed federal limits on the OTC sale of pseudoephedrine.
C. It made it illegal to sell alcohol to minors.
D. It required drugs to be dispensed with child-resistant bottle caps.

24. Drugs must be dispensed in child-resistant packaging according to the Poison Prevention Packaging Act (PPPA), but certain drugs are exempt from this requirement. Which one of the following drugs should not be dispensed in child-resistant packaging?

A. Zestril®
B. Valium®
C. Celexa®
D. Nitrostat®

25. Where can you find the expiration date of a prescription drug product?

A. On the manufacturer drug package label.
B. In the package insert.
C. Stamped directly on the tablet or capsule.
D. On the manufacturer's website.

26. Which reference would be used to determine whether a generic drug product is therapeutically equivalent to a brand drug product?

A. Red Book
B. Gold Standard Drug Database
C. Medi-Span
D. Orange Book

27. In the Orange Book, a generic drug that is therapeutically equivalent to a brand name drug would have a therapeutic equivalence (TE) rating beginning with which of the following letters?

A. A
B. B
C. C
D. X

28. Which information does not appear on an OTC package label?

A. Uses
B. Warnings
C. Directions
D. Off-Label Uses

29. Which of the following are not associated with HIPAA?

A. Protected health information (PHI).
B. The breach notification rule.
C. The principle of minimum necessary use and disclosure.
D. Coordination of benefits.

30. NDC numbers contain three segments. What does the first segment of an NDC number represent?

A. The identity the drug.
B. The package size.
C. The identity of the manufacturer.
D. None of the above.

31. A delayed-release tablet is most similar to which of the following?

A. Enteric-coated tablet
B. Controlled-release tablet
C. Extended-release capsule
D. Long-acting tablet

32. Which of the following is an indication for the OTC drug Azo® (phenazopyridine)?

A. Inflammation
B. Pinworms
C. Congestion
D. Urinary Pain

33. What dosage form must be shaken well prior to administration?

A. Elixir
B. Solution
C. Suspension
D. Cream

34. Which employee(s) is/are authorized to perform a drug utilization review (DUR)?

A. Pharmacy Technician
B. Certified Pharmacy Technician
C. Pharmacist
D. Cashier
E. Both B. and C.

35. Which of the following pieces of information is most useful in the event of a recall?

A. UPC Code
B. Expiration Date
C. Lot Number
D. Manufacturer Phone Number
E. None of the above

36. A patient drops off a prescription for an 84-day supply of Trinessa®, but her insurance will only pay for a 28-day supply. This is an example of a _________.

A. Coordination of benefits
B. Refill too soon rejection
C. Co-payment
D. Prior authorization
E. Plan limitation

37. Compared to brand name drugs, generic drugs often have which of the following characteristics?

A. Equal Quality
B. Equal Performance
C. Equal Safety
D. Lower Cost
E. All of the Above

38. Which of the following is an example of a brand name drug product?

A. Albuterol HFA
B. Lisinopril
C. Naproxen
D. Motrin

39. Match each brand name with the correct generic name.

A. Singulair®	I. Phenytoin
B. Desyrel®	II. Benzonatate
C. Dilantin®	III. Diazepam
D. Tessalon®	IV. Trazodone
E. Valium®	V. Montelukast

40. Which of the following is a sign of incompatibility in an IV admixture?

A. Bubbles
B. Precipitate formation
C. Cloudiness
D. Color change
E. All of the Above

41. Match each drug with the condition it is used to treat.

A. Meloxicam	I. Insomnia
B. Fexofenadine	II. Pain
C. Olmesartan	III. Inflammation
D. Fentanyl	IV. Hypertension
E. Zolpidem	V. Allergies

42. Which pregnancy category indicates that a drug should never be used during pregnancy?

A. Pregnancy Category A
B. Pregnancy Category B
C. Pregnancy Category C
D. Pregnancy Category D
E. Pregnancy Category X

43. Interpret the sig written on the prescription pictured below.

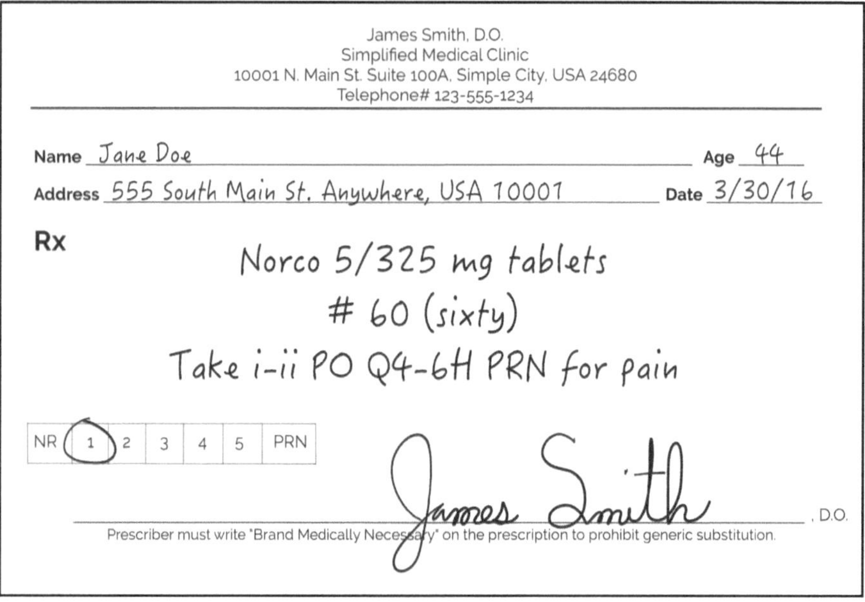
James Smith, D.O.
Simplified Medical Clinic
10001 N. Main St. Suite 100A, Simple City, USA 24680
Telephone# 123-555-1234

Name Jane Doe Age 44
Address 555 South Main St. Anywhere, USA 10001 Date 3/30/16

Rx
Norco 5/325 mg tablets
60 (sixty)
Take i-ii PO Q4-6H PRN for pain

NR	1	2	3	4	5	PRN

James Smith, D.O.
Prescriber must write "Brand Medically Necessary" on the prescription to prohibit generic substitution.

A. Take one and one-half milliliters by mouth every four to six hours as needed.
B. Take one to two milliliters every four to six hours as needed for pain.
C. Take one to two tablets by mouth every four to six hours as needed for pain.
D. Use as directed by physician.

44. Which piece of information is not commonly collected when creating a patient profile?

A. Date of Birth
B. Dental Insurance Information
C. Gender
D. Prescription Drug Insurance Information

45. Which of the following abbreviations should be avoided due to the potential for misinterpretation?

A. tab
B. mL
C. QD
D. kg

Use the prescription below to answer questions 46 – 47.

Simpletown Hospital
1111 N. Main St.
Anywhere, USA 54321
Telephone# 800-555-1111
Dr. Joe Smith, MD DEA#__________

Patient Name John Doe Date 10/12/2016

Address 222 North Main St. Sumwhere, USA 65432 DOB 01/07/1976

Rx

BuPROPion XL 300 mg

#30 tablets

Take one tablet by mouth once daily

2 Refills

J. Smith M.D.

Product Selection Permitted

Dispense as Written

46. How has Dr. Joe Smith implemented safety strategies for this prescription?

A. Dr. Smith used tall man lettering.
B. Dr. Smith did not use any error-prone abbreviations.
C. Dr. Smith did not use trailing zeros.
D. All of the above.

47. What is bupropion used to treat?

A. Depression
B. Hypertension
C. ADHD
D. Rabies

48. What does the sig code AU stand for?

A. Left eye
B. Both eyes
C. Left ear
D. Both ears
E. Australia

49. When creating or updating a patient profile, how should you respond if the patient refuses to disclose the information requested?

A. Document the refusal in the patient profile.
B. Argue with the patient.
C. Call the patient's spouse to obtain the information.
D. All of the Above.

Use the prescription below to answer questions 50 – 52.

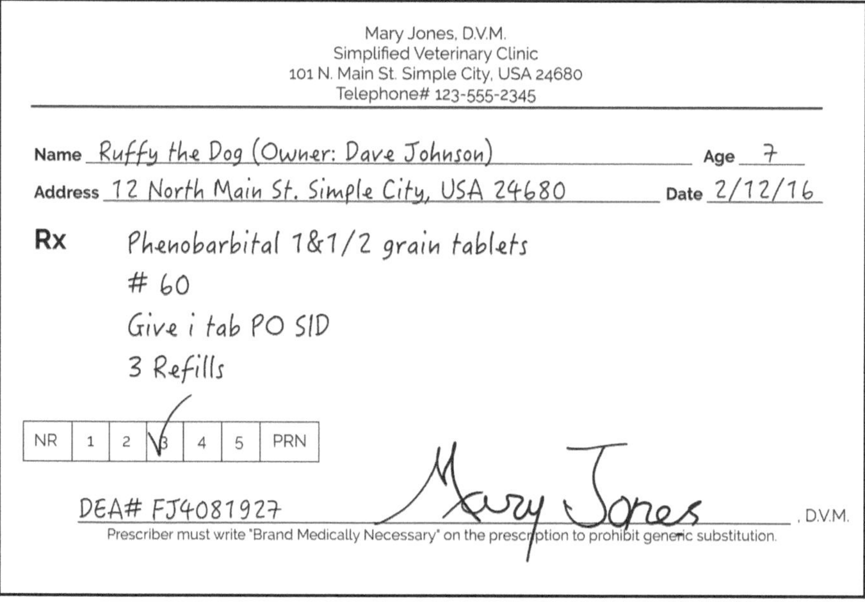

Mary Jones, D.V.M.
Simplified Veterinary Clinic
101 N. Main St. Simple City, USA 24680
Telephone# 123-555-2345

Name Ruffy the Dog (Owner: Dave Johnson) Age 7
Address 12 North Main St. Simple City, USA 24680 Date 2/12/16

Rx Phenobarbital 1&1/2 grain tablets
60
Give i tab PO SID
3 Refills

NR	1	2	3 ✓	4	5	PRN

DEA# FJ4081927 Mary Jones, D.V.M.

Prescriber must write "Brand Medically Necessary" on the prescription to prohibit generic substitution.

50. The prescription is written for 60 tablets of 1 ½ grain Phenobarbital. The pharmacy has four different strengths of Phenobarbital in stock. Which strength should be dispensed to fill Ruffy's prescription?

A. 16.2 mg
B. 32.4 mg
C. 64.8 mg
D. 97.2 mg

51. According to the prescription, how many times a day should Ruffy receive a dose?

A. Once daily
B. Twice daily
C. Four times daily
D. Every other day

52. What is wrong with the DEA number on the prescription written by Mary Jones, DVM?

A. DEA numbers for veterinarians cannot begin with the letter "F."
B. DEA number on the prescription must be typed (cannot be handwritten).
C. Valid DEA numbers contain 2 letters followed by an 8-digit number.
D. Nothing is wrong with the veterinarian's DEA number.

53. Federal law indicates that prescription records must be kept for 2 years, but the state law where you work indicates that prescription records must be kept for 3 years. The records should be kept for ________.

A. 2 years
B. 2 & ½ years
C. 3 years
D. 4 years
E. None of the above

54. HydrALAzine and HydrOXYzine are examples of ________________________.

A. Allergy medications
B. Brand name medications
C. Separating inventory
D. Look-alike/sound-alike medications
E. Drug regimen reviews

55. In which situation is it appropriate to indicate a DAW 7 code when dispensing the brand name of a drug?

A. When the prescriber writes "brand medically necessary" on the prescription.
B. When law mandates that the brand product be dispensed.
C. When the patient requests the brand name drug.
D. When substitution is permitted, but the generic version is unavailable.

56. What are the four numbers that are needed to submit a claim to a prescription drug insurance company?

A. BIN, Group Number, ID Number, Telephone Number
B. PCN, Group Number, Telephone Number, Employer ID
C. ID Number, Employer ID, Group Number, DEA Number
D. BIN, PCN, Group Number, ID Number

57. What are auxiliary labels used for?

A. To display the number of refills remaining on a prescription.
B. To provide additional information for proper use and storage of a medication.
C. To create a tamper-evident seal over the lid of a prescription bottle.
D. To provide the patient with a toll-free number where a pharmacist can be reached.

58. When is it necessary to shake a drug suspension or emulsion?

A. As soon as the drug order is received by the pharmacy.
B. Immediately prior to measuring quantities for dispensing.
C. Immediately prior to administration.
D. Both B & C

59. What is the purpose of tall man lettering?

A. To emphasize the spelling differences between medications with similar names.
B. To standardize the font size for medication names as they appear on stock bottles.
C. To make it easier to separate inventory.
D. To eliminate the need for NDC numbers.
E. None of the above.

60. Which of the following would not help avoid errors?

A. Promoting patient counseling.
B. Reading back verbal prescription orders.
C. Using leading zeros when writing numbers with values less than one.
D. Using trailing zeros when writing numbers with values greater than one.

61. Which of the following medications should be dispensed in the original packaging?

A. Celexa® (Citalopram)
B. Pradaxa® (Dabigatran)
C. Nitrostat® (Nitroglycerin)
D. Zestril® (Lisinopril)
E. Both B & C

62. You are in the clean room and an order comes in for norepinephrine 10 mg in 250 mL of D5W. How many vials of norepinephrine will you need to open if it comes in 4 mg/4 mL vials?

A. 1 vial
B. 2 vials
C. 3 vials
D. 4 vials
E. 2.5 vials

63. You receive an order for 90 mL of lidocaine 4% nasal spray. You will use normal saline solution and 10% lidocaine solution to compound this prescription. How much 10% lidocaine solution will be needed?

A. 18 mL
B. 27 mL
C. 36 mL
D. 45 mL
E. 54 mL

64. You are using a class A prescription balance with a sensitivity requirement of 6 mg. Using this balance, you can measure 300 mg of a substance within ___ % error.

A. 1
B. 2
C. 3
D. 4
E. 5

65. A patient presents a prescription for 450 milliliters of allopurinol 40 mg/mL oral suspension. Allopurinol is available from the manufacturer in an oral tablet form only. Using allopurinol 100 mg tablets, how many tablets will you need to pulverize and triturate to compound this prescription?

A. 90 tablets
B. 100 tablets
C. 125 tablets
D. 180 tablets
E. 250 tablets

66. The pharmacist wants the refrigerator temperature to be set to 6°C. What is this temperature in degrees Fahrenheit?

A. 0°F
B. 32°F
C. 35°F
D. 43°F
E. 100°F

67. If a solution of ampicillin is being infused at the rate of 60 drops per minute, how long will it take to infuse 100 milliliters if the administration set delivers 20 drops per milliliter?

A. 23 minutes
B. 25minutes
C. 30 minutes
D. 33 minutes
E. 35 minutes

68. Tanya weighs 210 pounds and has a life-threatening fungal infection. Her physician prescribes a 0.3 mg/kg dose of amphotericin B. How many micrograms of amphotericin B should Tanya receive?

A. 29 mg
B. 63 mg
C. 29,000 mcg
D. 63,000 mcg
E. 33 mg

69. The dose of experimental drug DH671244 is 55 mg/m^2 every 8 hours. How many milligrams of DH671244 should be given over the course of 24 hours for a male patient that is exactly 6 feet tall and weighs 240 pounds?

A. 190 mg
B. 280 mg
C. 390 mg
D. 460 mg
E. 530 mg

70. Which of the following statements is correct regarding scored tablets?

A. Scored tablets should never be split or cut.
B. Scored tablets are designed for sublingual administration.
C. Scored tablets always have a circular shape.
D. Scored tablets are designed to be easily split into fractions.
E. Scored tablets will not dissolve until they reach the small intestine.

71. Which of the following is a type of insurance plan?

A. NDC
B. PBM
C. CMS
D. PPE
E. PPO

72. If the normal adult dose of clindamycin is 300 mg, then what is the dose for a 4-year-old patient that weighs 60 pounds? (Calculate the dose using Clark's Rule)

A. 55 mg
B. 100 mg
C. 110 mg
D. 120 mg
E. 165 mg

73. A prescription is written for prednisone 10 mg tablets with instructions to take 4 tablets daily for 2 days, then 3 tablets daily for 2 days, then 2 tablets daily for 2 days, then 1 tablet daily for 2 days, then ½ tablet daily for 2 days, then stop. How many tablets will you need to dispense?

A. 18 tablets
B. 21 tablets
C. 24 tablets
D. 27 tablets
E. 30 tablets

74. A prescription is written for 60 tablets of Wellbutrin XL 150 mg with instructions for the patient to take 1 tablet by mouth once daily for 8 days and then take 2 tablets by mouth once daily thereafter. What is the days' supply?

A. 27 days
B. 30 days
C. 33 days
D. 34 days
E. 38 days

75. According to the manufacturer, Travatan Z® eye drops should be stored at or between 2 – 25°C. Which of the following environments would be acceptable?

A. A cold environment
B. A cool environment
C. A room temperature environment
D. Both B. and C.
E. All of the above

76. Which of the following could be an example of an NDC number?

A. 0093-0437-01
B. 01232-543-1
C. 9678-234-09
D. 00781-5824-100
E. All of the Above

77. When handling needles (e.g. when compounding sterile products for infusion), it is important to...

A. Always recap the needle after it has been used.
B. Never recap the needle after it has been used.
C. Place the used needle in a red sharps container.
D. Both A. and C.
E. Both B. and C.

78. When selecting a filter for Total Nutrient Admixtures (TNAs), which contain emulsified fat droplets, what is the optimal pore size?

A. 1 centimeter
B. 0.5 microns
C. 0.22 microns
D. 1.2 microns
E. None of the above

79. In what order should the following clean room garb be donned? (Number from first to last)

___ Shoe Covers
___ Gloves
___ Gown
___ Face Mask
___ Hair Cover

80. A 1000-tablet bottle of metformin 500 mg is repackaged into unit dose packages. Assuming the expiration date printed on the stock bottle label is at least two (2) years from today, what is the maximum beyond-use date for the repackaged doses if no stability tests are conducted?

A. 1 month
B. 3 months
C. 6 months
D. 2 years

81. Your pharmacy purchases 30-tablet bottles of citalopram 20 mg from a distributor at the price of $7.45/bottle. What is the retail cost of each bottle if the pharmacy has a 29% markup and a $9 dispensing fee?

A. $16.89
B. $18.61
C. $20.32
D. $23.40

82. Which of the following parenteral administration routes requires the use of sterile, preservative-free (PF) ingredients?

A. Intravenous
B. Epidural
C. Intradermal
D. Subcutaneous

Use the prescription below to answer questions 83 – 85.

Dr. James Smith
1000 Main St. Suite B
Anytown, USA 10001

NPI# 10000000001 Telephone# 800-555-0000 DEA#__________

Patient Name Joe Smotly Date 11/14/2016

Address 333 Main St. Anytown, USA 10001 DOB 01/02/1977

Rx

Doxycycline 100 mg

#14

Take i PO Q12H x 7 days

No Refills

J. Smith M.D.

Product Selection Permitted Dispense as Written

83. What instructions should appear on the label of Mr. Smotly's prescription?

   A. Take one tablet by mouth every 12 hours for 7 days.
   B. Apply 100 mg to the oral cavity for 12 hours every 7 days.
   C. Give one tablet to your dog "Po" every 12 hours for 7 days.
   D. Take as directed.

84. If Mr. Smotly begins to feel better after taking doxycycline for 3 days, should he stop taking the medication?

   A. Yes, to reduce the chance of side effects.
   B. No, a patient must take an antibiotic for years to achieve the optimal result.
   C. Yes, to reduce the chance of drug interactions.
   D. No, by discontinuing antibiotics early, the bacteria causing the infection can develop resistance to the treatment and come back even stronger.

85. The patient does not object to receiving the generic form of Coumadin®, and you have a generic in stock. When billing his insurance company for this prescription, which DAW code will you select?

A. DAW 0
B. DAW 1
C. DAW 2
D. DAW 6

86. Which term refers to the process of reducing the particle size of a powder?

A. Trituration
B. Geometric dilution
C. Aseptic technique
D. Rule of hand

87. Which of the following resources provides guidance on good compounding practices for non-sterile compounded drug products?

A. The Orange Book
B. USP Chapter 795
C. The Package Insert
D. USP Chapter 797

88. You receive a prescription order for a 5-year-old patient. The prescription is for ibuprofen 100 mg/5 mL suspension with instructions to take 10 mL by mouth every 6 hours. The maximum daily dose of ibuprofen for a patient age 6 months to 12 years is 40 mg/kg/day. If the patient weighs 44 pounds, what is the maximum daily dose for this patient? Is the prescribed daily dose equal to or less than the maximum daily dose?

A. 440 mg; No
B. 200 mg; Yes
C. 800 mg; Yes
D. 1,760 mg; No

89. Which of the following activities should take place in a buffer area?

A. Removing personal protective equipment.
B. Eating snacks.
C. Recapping needles.
D. Sterile compounding.

90. Which of the following factors do not typically have a negative effect on drug stability?

A. Sunlight
B. Darkness
C. Humidity
D. Heat

91. Cheratussin® DAC contains 2.1% (v/v) alcohol. How many milliliters of alcohol are in one 16-ounce bottle (473 mL)?

A. 2.1 mL
B. 1 tsp
C. 9.9 mL
D. 20 tsp

92. When in continuous use, a laminar airflow hood should be cleaned with 70% isopropyl alcohol every ______.

A. 30 minutes
B. 1 hour
C. 2 hours
D. 6 hours

93. Which filter pore size is most effective for filtering out microorganisms (e.g. bacteria, fungi)?

A. 0.22 microns
B. 0.3 microns
C. 0.5 microns
D. 1.2 microns

94. How many pairs of disposable gloves should be worn by an individual cleaning up a hazardous drug spill?

A. 1 pair
B. 2 pairs
C. 3 pairs
D. 4 pairs

95. A patient receives a prescription for Vitamin D_2 (ergocalciferol) 50,000 unit capsules with instructions to take one capsule by mouth once weekly. What is the days' supply for 12 capsules?

A. 77 days
B. 78 days
C. 84 days
D. 90 days

96. A patient is receiving a 100-mL infusion of metronidazole 500 mg over the course of 30 minutes. If the administration set delivers 20 drops/mL, what is the drip rate for the infusion?

A. 33 drops/minute
B. 50 drops/minute
C. 67 drops/minute
D. 100 drops/minute

97. Jane walks into your pharmacy to purchase pen needles for her insulin pens. Jane says that she wants the thinnest ½ inch-long needle you have. If the following needle sizes represent what you have in stock, which size should you give her?

A. 29 gauge, 12.7 millimeters
B. 31 gauge, 12.7 millimeters
C. 30 gauge, 8 millimeters
D. 32 gauge, 8 millimeters

98. If C-III, C-IV, and C-V controlled substance prescription records are stored in the same file with non-controlled substance prescription records, what mark must appear on the lower right corner of the controlled substance prescription?

A. In blue ink, a Roman numeral indicating the schedule of the prescribed controlled substance.
B. In black ink, the letters "CS" at least 1-½ inches high.
C. In red ink, the letter "C" at least 1 inch high.
D. In indelible ink, the initials of the dispensing pharmacist at least 2 inches high.

99. Which drug combination could result in a dangerous drug-drug interaction?

A. Prinivil® + Tenormin®
B. Pravachol® + Glucotrol®
C. Lovenox® + Delsym®
D. Viagra® + Nitrostat®

100. Based on the definition of each word part, what does the term "arthritis" mean?

A. Bone disease
B. Shoulder pain
C. Joint inflammation
D. Mental condition

101. What are the four parts of a prescription sig?

A. Patient's name, quantity, number of refills, expiration date
B. Action word, quantity with units, route of administration, dosing frequency
C. Patient's name, address, date of birth, date issued
D. Verb, noun, adjective, noun

102. Typically, how long does it take for an insurance company to process a prior authorization?

A. A few hours
B. A few days
C. A few weeks
D. A few months

103. Which of the following statements is true regarding the practice of compounding?

A. A compounded drug product may contain up to one ingredient that has been deemed unsafe.
B. A compounded drug product may be a copy of a commercially available FDA-approved drug product.
C. Compounding can take place under the supervision of a registered pharmaceutical manufacturer.
D. A drug product can only be compounded after receiving an individual, patient-specific prescription order, or in anticipation of receiving a patient-specific prescription order based on an established prescribing pattern.

104. Which of the following should not be worn in a clean room/buffer area?

A. Hair cover
B. Artificial nails
C. Shoe covers
D. None of the above

105. The quantity for a prescription for diphenhydramine 12.5 mg/5 mL elixir is written by the prescriber as "CXX milliliters." How many ounces of the elixir should you dispense? (Calculate your answer based on a conversion factor of 30 mL per ounce)

A. 2 ounces
B. 4 ounces
C. 6 ounces
D. 8 ounces

106. Oxycodone is a __________ controlled substance.

A. Schedule II
B. Schedule III
C. Schedule IV
D. Schedule V

107. What agency or organization is responsible for the administration of Medicare?

A. DEA
B. FDA
C. CMS
D. ISMP

108. Sandra has prescription drug insurance, but she has never used it. Which of the following payments has Sandra probably made to her insurance company?

A. Premium
B. Deductible
C. Co-payment
D. All of the above
E. None of the above

109. What are "analgesics?"

A. Drugs for bacterial infections
B. Drugs for high blood pressure
C. Drugs for pain
D. Drugs for dementia

110. Which one of the following insulin formulations is available over-the-counter (OTC)?

A. Lantus
B. Novolin 70/30
C. Levemir
D. Humalog

111. Which one of the following products reverses the effect of warfarin?

A. Vitamin K
B. Aspirin
C. Senna
D. Metformin

112. How long is a vial of insulin stable at room temperature?

A. 14 days
B. 28 days
C. 30 days
D. 180 days

113. Match each brand name with its associated generic name.

A. Toprol XL®	I. Carbamazepine
B. Lamisil®	II. Terbinafine
C. Ritalin®	III. Metoprolol (ER)
D. Apresoline®	IV. Methylphenidate
E. Tegretol®	V. Hydralazine

114. A patient presents a prescription for amoxicillin 500 mg capsules with instructions to take 500 mg by mouth every 6 hours for 14 days. How many capsules should you dispense?

A. 42 capsules
B. 56 capsules
C. 68 capsules
D. 72 capsules
E. Not enough information

115. Calcium has a molecular weight of 40 and a valence of 2. Given this information, what is the mass (in milligrams) of 12 mEq of calcium?

A. 120 mEq
B. 160 mEq
C. 200 mEq
D. 240 mEq

116. What is the role of the Drug Enforcement Administration (DEA)?

A. Enforce occupational health laws.
B. Regulate large-scale compounding facilities.
C. Enforce federal controlled substance laws.
D. Regulate OTC drug advertising.

117. Which of the following is a task that cannot be completed by a pharmacy technician?

A. Dispose of expired drug products.
B. Deliver completed/filled prescriptions.
C. Place orders for out of stock medications.
D. Evaluate prescriptions for drug interactions.

Use the prescription below to answer questions 118 – 119.

Simpletown Hospital
1111 N. Main St.
Anywhere, USA 54321
Telephone# 800-555-1111
Dr. Joe Smith, MD DEA#______________

Patient Name John Doe Date 10/12/2016

Address 222 North Main St. Sumwhere, USA 65432 DOB 01/07/1976

Rx

1:1 Mixture of Eucerin Cream & Triamcinolone 0.5% Ointment

Dispense 1-pound jar

AAA BID PRN for itchy rash

NR

J. Smith M.D.

Product Selection Permitted Dispense as Written

118. How many grams of each ingredient are needed to compound the prescription?

   A. 500 g of Eucerin® cream and 500 g of triamcinolone 0.5% ointment
   B. 227 g of Eucerin® cream and 227 g of triamcinolone 0.5% ointment
   C. 500 g of Eucerin® cream and 500 g of triamcinolone 1% ointment
   D. 254 g of Eucerin® cream and 254 g of triamcinolone 1% ointment
   E. 0.5 kg of Eucerin® cream and 0.5 kg of triamcinolone 1% ointment

119. What should the instructions say on the prescription label?

   A. Apply all amounts three times daily as directed for itchy rash
   B. Apply to affected area twice daily as needed for itchy rash
   C. Apply all amounts once daily for itchy rash
   D. Apply to affected area four times daily as needed for itchy rash

120. What is the minimum age for purchasing OTC Schedule V controlled substances?

   A. 12 years old
   B. 16 years old
   C. 18 years old
   D. 21 years old

PRACTICE EXAM ANSWER KEY

1. C. 143 lbs

$$65 \text{ kg} \times \frac{2.2 \text{ lb}}{\text{kg}} = 143 \text{ lb}$$

2. C. September 30, 2015

To review this topic, see "Lot Numbers and Expiration Dates" on page 29.

3. D. Levetiracetam

BRAND NAME	GENERIC NAME
Prevacid®	Lansoprazole
Lamictal®	Lamotrigine
Atrovent®	Ipratropium
Keppra®	Levetiracetam

4. D. Recommending an OTC medication for a patient.

To review this topic, see page 23.

5. C. Class III

There are three (3) classes of FDA recalls: class I, class II, and class III. The class I recall is the most severe – serious adverse health consequences, up to and including death, are possible. The class III recall is the least severe – the product is unlikely to cause any adverse health consequences.

6. D. Type a prescription label.

To review the Pharmacy Technician's Role and Function, see pages 23 – 24.

7. C. Assist the pharmacist.

To review this topic, see page 23.

8. B. Yellow sharps container

	Red Container	Yellow Container	Black Container
Standard Sharps Waste	✓		
Sharps Waste with Hazardous Drug Residue		✓	
Bulk Hazardous Drug Waste			✓

9. D. To ensure that drugs closer to expiration are dispensed first.

To review Basic Inventory Management, see page 28.

10. B. DEA

AGENCY	ROLE
FDA	Enforces drug manufacturing laws. Regulates prescription drug advertising and large-scale compounding.
DEA	Enforces the federal Controlled Substances Act (CSA). Classifies controlled substances.
OSHA	Enforces employee health and safety laws.
FTC	Regulates OTC drug, medical device, cosmetic, and food advertising.

11. B. Schedule II

SCHEDULE	MEDICAL USES	ABUSE POTENTIAL	DEPENDENCE POTENTIAL
C-I	No	High	High
C-II	Yes	High	High
C-III	Yes	Moderate	Moderate-Low
C-IV	Yes	Mild	Mild
C-V	Yes	Low	Low

12. B. No

When asked whether or not a DEA number is valid, you must apply the 4-step process outlined on page 44. When you take the DEA number shown on the prescription (AS2389518) and apply the 4-step verification process, you see that the last digit of the DEA number should be "1;" however, the last digit of this prescriber's DEA number is "8." For that reason, the DEA number is not valid.

13. B. 3.6 grams

SUMMARY OF PSEUDOEPHEDRINE SALES LIMITS (PER CUSTOMER)

24-HOUR LIMIT (RETAIL OR MAIL ORDER)	30-DAY LIMIT (RETAIL)	30-DAY LIMIT (MAIL ORDER)
3.6 grams	9 grams	7.5 grams

To review OTC Pseudoephedrine Sales, see page 42.

14. B. DEA Form 222

FORM	PURPOSE
DEA Form 41	To report to the DEA the destruction of controlled substances
DEA Form 106	To report to the DEA the theft or loss of controlled substances.
DEA Form 222	To order (or to document the transfer of) Schedule I or Schedule II controlled substances

To review this topic further, see "DEA Forms" on page 43.

15. D. Both A & C.

All hydrocodone combination products are Schedule II controlled substances. According to federal law, refills are prohibited for all Schedule II controlled substances. Additionally, all prescriptions for controlled substances must include the prescriber's DEA number. There are no federal laws or rules that require any type of patient identification number to appear on the face of a prescription.

16. D. 5-day supply; DAW 0.

Since the prescriber did not write "Brand Name Medically Necessary" on the prescription and the patient did not request the brand name product, the DAW code is "0." The days' supply should always be calculated under the assumption that the patient will use the maximum amount of medication in accordance with the prescribed instructions. In this case, the maximum amount is 2 tablets every 4 hours, which is equal to 12 tablets per day. At this point, simple multiplication will tell us how many days the prescription should last:

$$60 \text{ tablets} \times \frac{\text{day}}{12 \text{ tablets}} = 5 \text{ days}$$

See pages 195 – 199 to review days' supply calculations and pages 141 – 142 to review DAW codes.

17. B. Up to 5 refills.

The federal Controlled Substances Act limits the number of refills on a C-III or C-IV controlled substance to a maximum of 5 refills within 6 months. To review the summary of the federal Controlled Substances Act requirements, see page 39.

18. C. Ambien®

Ambien® (zolpidem) is a Schedule IV controlled substance. To review controlled substances, see pages 32 – 35.

19. B. Letter X

To review this topic, see the note at the bottom of page 45.

20. B. NPI Number

ID NUMBER	PURPOSE
DEA Number	Required to issue prescriptions for controlled substances
NPI Number	Required for insurance claim submission/billing
UPIN	No longer in use – has been replaced by the NPI number

To review the section on prescriber identification numbers, see page 49.

21. D. To protect the privacy of patient health information.

To review this topic, see “Health Insurance Portability & Accountability Act (HIPAA)” on page 46.

22. B. Nurse Practitioner

To review the section on prescribing authority, see page 48.

23. D. It required drugs to be dispensed with child-resistant bottle caps.

To review the details of this law, see page 50.

24. D. Nitrostat®

To review the details of this law, see page 50.

25. A. On the manufacturer drug package label.

To review this information, see pages 52 – 54.

26. D. Orange Book

To review the section on generic substitution and the Orange Book, see page 47.

27. A. A

To review the section on generic substitution and the Orange Book, see page 47.

28. D. Off-Label Uses

To review the section on OTC drug package labels, see page 55. To review the definition of “off-label” see page 19.

29. D. Coordination of benefits.

To review HIPAA, see page 46. To review coordination of benefits, see page 151.

30. C. The identity of the manufacturer.

NDC SEGMENT	PURPOSE
#1 (5 digits)	Identifies the manufacturer
#2 (4 digits)	Identifies the product
#3 (2 digits)	Identifies the package size (usually)

To review the section on NDC numbers, see page 128.

31. A. Enteric-coated tablet

To review the section on modified-release dosage forms, see page 61.

32. D. Urinary Pain

To review the top 45 OTC drugs, see pages 121 – 122.

33. C. Suspension

To review liquid dosage forms, see page 58.

34. C. Pharmacist

To review this topic, see page 23.

35. C. Lot Number

To review lot numbers, see page 29.

36. E. Plan limitation

To review prescription drug insurance, see pages 147 –151.

37. E. All of the Above

To review generic substitution, see page 47.

38. D. Motrin

To review the top 200 prescription drugs, see pages 116 – 120.

39. A. Singulair® - V. Montelukast
B. Desyrel® - IV. Trazodone
C. Dilantin® - I. Phenytoin
D. Tessalon® - II. Benzonatate
E. Valium® - III. Diazepam

To review the top 200 prescription drugs, see pages 116 – 120.

40. E. All of the Above

To review the signs of incompatibility, see page 223.

41. A. Meloxicam - III. Inflammation
B. Fexofenadine - V. Allergies
C. Olmesartan - IV. Hypertension
D. Fentanyl - II. Pain
E. Zolpidem - I. Insomnia

To review the top 200 prescription drugs, see pages 116 – 120.

42. E. Pregnancy Category X

To review the subject of pregnancy categories, see the key term on page 20.

43. C. Take one to two tablets by mouth every four to six hours as needed for pain.

To review sig codes, see pages 131 – 135.

44. B. Dental Insurance Information

To review patient profiles, see page 130.

45. C. QD

To review error prone abbreviations, see page 139.

46. D. All of the above.

To review methods for avoiding errors, see pages 137 – 140.

47. A. Depression

To review the top 200 prescription drugs, see pages 116 – 120.

48. D. Both ears

SIG CODE	MEANING
AD	right ear
AS	left ear
AU	both ears
OD	right eye
OS	left eye
OU	both eyes

To review sig codes, see pages 131 – 135.

49. A. Document the refusal in the patient's profile.

To review patient profiles, see page 130.

50. D. 97.2 mg

$$1.5 \text{ grains} \times \frac{64.8 \text{ mg}}{\text{grain}} = 97.2 \text{ mg}$$

To review must-know conversion factors, see page 163.

51. A. Once daily

SID is a sig code used almost exclusively by veterinarians. It has the same meaning as QD (once daily). To review sig codes, see pages 131 – 135.

52. D. Nothing is wrong with the veterinarian's DEA number.

To review the 4-step DEA number verification process, see page 44.

53. C. 3 years

You do not need to know specific state laws for the ExCPT exam, but you do need to know this simple rule – when federal and state laws differ, the more stringent law applies.

54. D. Look-alike/sound-alike medications

To review look-alike/sound-alike medications, see page 137.

55. B. When law mandates that the brand product be dispensed.

To review DAW codes, see pages 141 – 142.

56. D. BIN, PCN, Group Number, ID Number

To review prescription drug insurance, see page 147.

57. B. To provide additional information for proper use and storage of a medication.

To review the topic of auxiliary labels, see page 143.

58. D. Both B & C

To review liquid dosage forms, see page 58.

59. A. To emphasize the spelling differences between medications with similar names.

To review tall man lettering, see page 137.

60. D. Using trailing zeros when writing numbers with values greater than one.

Never use trailing zeros! To review this subject, see page 138.

61. E. Both B & C

DRUG PRODUCT	SPECIAL STORAGE REQUIREMENT
Nitrostat® (Nitroglycerin Sublingual Tablets)	Do not remove tablets from original container. Nitroglycerin is a volatile substance that quickly converts from solid to gas. When stored outside of the original container, the nitroglycerin will evaporate from the tablet. For this reason, it is important to keep nitroglycerin tablets tightly sealed in the original container (usually a small glass vial with metal lid).
Pradaxa® (Dabigatran Oral Capsules)	Pradaxa® is available in a bottle or blister packs. For the bottle, it is important not to remove the capsules from from their original container until immediately prior to use. The drug is quickly destroyed by humidity in the air. The Pradaxa® bottle is equipped with a special cap that contains a desiccant (drying agent). Once the bottle is opened, the capsules inside expire after 4 months. For the blister packs, do not remove a capsule from the blister pack until immediately prior to use.

To review storage requirements, see pages 144 – 146.

62. C. 3 vials

The solution involves unit conversion with a tricky twist. You know that 10 mg of norepinephrine are needed to prepare the order, and one vial contains 4 mg of norepinephrine. You will need a volume equal to 2.5 vials to prepare the order; however, the question asks how many vials you would need to puncture/open to prepare this order. You would need to open 3 vials to obtain that volume. When taking the ExCPT exam, pay close attention to the way each question is worded. Some of the questions may be trickier than they first appear.

$$10 \text{ mg} \times \frac{\text{vial}}{4 \text{ mg}} = 2.5 \text{ vials} \therefore 3 \text{ vials}$$

63. C. 36 mL

This is an alligation problem.

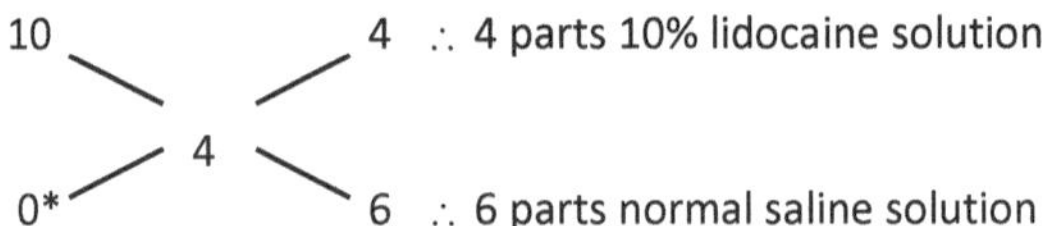

* Normal saline solution contains zero percent lidocaine.

This compound will consist of 10 parts (4 parts 10 % lidocaine solution and 6 parts normal saline solution). In other words, four-tenths (4/10) of the 90 mL prescription will be composed of the 10% lidocaine solution and the other six-tenths (6/10) will be composed of normal saline solution (i.e. 0% lidocaine solution).

$$\frac{90 \text{ mL}}{10 \text{ parts}} \times \frac{4 \text{ parts of 10\% Lidocaine}}{1} = 36 \text{ mL of 10\% Lidocaine}$$

To review alligation, see pages 185 – 189.

64. B. 2

If you know the sensitivity requirement of the balance (6 mg in this case) and the weight of a substance being measured (300 mg), you can calculate the percent error using the following equation:

$$\% \text{ Error} = \frac{\text{Sensitivity Requirement}}{\text{Measured Weight}} \times 100\% = \frac{6 \text{ mg}}{300 \text{ mg}} \times 100\% = 2\%$$

To review percent error, see pages 192 – 194. To memorize the common pharmacy math equations, see Appendix A on page 277.

65. D. 180 tablets

To solve this problem, the first thing you must do is determine how many milligrams of allopurinol are needed to compound the entire prescription. This is a simple, one-step multiplication problem:

$$450 \text{ mL} \times \frac{40 \text{ mg}}{\text{mL}} = 18{,}000 \text{ mg}$$

Since we know there are 100 milligrams of allopurinol in each tablet, the next step is just as easy:

$$18{,}000 \text{ mg} \times \frac{\text{tablet}}{100 \text{ mg}} = 180 \text{ tablets}$$

66. D. 43°F

$$°\text{F} = \left(\frac{9}{5} \times °\text{C}\right) + 32$$

67. D. 33 minutes

$$100 \text{ mL} \times \frac{20 \text{ drops}}{\text{mL}} \times \frac{\text{minute}}{60 \text{ drops}} = 33 \text{ minutes}$$

68. C. 29,000 mcg

Pay close attention to the units. This question specifically asked for an answer in micrograms.

$$210 \text{ lb} \times \frac{\text{kg}}{2.2 \text{ lb}} \times \frac{0.3 \text{ mg}}{\text{kg}} \times \frac{1{,}000 \text{ mcg}}{\text{mg}} = 28{,}636 \text{ mcg} \therefore 29{,}000 \text{ mcg}$$

69. C. 390 mg

The solution to this problem involves multiple steps. First, you need to calculate the patient's body surface area (BSA). To calculate BSA, you must convert height to centimeters and weight to kilograms. Once you determine the patient's BSA, multiply it by 55 mg/m^2 to calculate the dose. Finally, you must multiply the dose by 3 since the patient will receive 1 dose every 8 hours and the question asks how many milligrams will be given in a 24-hour period.

To review BSA dosing, see page 201.

70. D. Scored tablets are designed to be easily split into fractions.

To review this topic, see page 59.

71. E. PPO

To review this topic, see pages 148.

72. D. 120 mg

$$\text{Child Dose} = \frac{60 \text{ lb}}{150 \text{ lb}} \times 300 \text{ mg} = 120 \text{ mg}$$

To review pediatric dosing equations, see pages 202 – 204.

73. B. 21 tablets

$$\left(\frac{4 \text{ tablets}}{\text{day}} \times 2 \text{ days}\right) + \left(\frac{3 \text{ tablets}}{\text{day}} \times 2 \text{ days}\right) + \left(\frac{2 \text{ tablets}}{\text{day}} \times 2 \text{ days}\right)$$

$$+ \left(\frac{1 \text{ tablet}}{\text{day}} \times 2 \text{ days}\right) + \left(\frac{0.5 \text{ tablet}}{\text{day}} \times 2 \text{ days}\right)$$

$$= 21 \text{ tablets}$$

74. D. 34 days

After the first 8 days of therapy, the patient will have 52 tablets remaining. Those 52 tablets will be sufficient to last 26 days (52 divided by 2, since the patient takes 2 tablets daily; see math below). So, the first 8 tablets last 8 days and the remaining 52 tablets will last 26 days. Then it is simple addition, 8 days + 26 days = 34 days.

$$\text{For the first 8 days:} \quad 8 \text{ tablets} \times \frac{\text{day}}{1 \text{ tablet}} = 8 \text{ days}$$

$$\text{After the first 8 days:} \quad 52 \text{ tablets} \times \frac{\text{day}}{2 \text{ tablets}} = 26 \text{ days}$$

75. E. All of the above

TEMPERATURE RANGES	
Cold	2°C to 8°C (36°F to 46°F)
Cool	8°C to 15°C (46°F to 59°F)
Room Temperature	20°C to 25°C (68°F to 77°F)

All of these environments fall within the manufacturer's recommended range.

76. A. 0093-0437-01

NDC numbers consist of 11 digits (a 5-digit segment to identify the manufacturer, a 4-digit segment to identify the drug product, and a 2-digit segment that is usually used to identify the package size). In most cases, when a segment contains one or more leading zeros, one of the leading zeros will be omitted. For instance, 00093-0437-01 would be expressed in any one of the following three ways:

0093-0437-01
00093-437-01
00093-0437-1

77. E. Both B. and C.

It is never a good idea to recap a needle. Recapping increases the chance of a needle stick injury. Red sharps containers are the standard waste disposal containers for medical needles and sharp objects.

78. D. 1.2 microns

1.2 micron pores are large enough to allow the fat droplets to pass through the filter without clogging it. Smaller pores would be clogged by the fat droplets, and larger pores would allow harmful fungi and particles to pass through the filter. To review this topic, see pages 220.

79. 1 Shoe Covers
2 Hair Cover
3 Face Mask
4 Gown
5 Gloves

In general, you want to put on your clean room garb in the order of dirtiest to cleanest (shoes are assumed to be the dirtiest and washed hands are considered to be the cleanest).

To review this topic, see pages 213 – 214.

80. C. 6 months

To review medication repackaging, see page 212.

81. B. $18.61

Retail Cost = [AWP x (1 + Markup*)] + Dispensing Fee
*Markup expressed as a decimal

Retail Cost = [$7.45 x (1 + 0.29)] + $9 = $18.61

To review drug pricing, see pages 208 – 211.

82. B. Epidural

To review parenteral administration routes, see pages 225 – 226.

83. A. Take one tablet by mouth every 12 hours for 7 days.

To review sig codes, see pages 131 – 135.

84. D. No, by discontinuing antibiotics early, the bacteria causing the infection can develop resistance to the treatment and come back even stronger.

85. A. DAW 0

To review DAW codes, see pages 141 – 142.

86. A. Trituration

To review non-sterile compounding, see pages 190 – 194.

87. B. USP Chapter 795

To review non-sterile compounding, see pages 190 – 194.

88. C. 800 mg; Yes

$$\text{Maximum Daily Dose: } 44\text{ lb} \times \frac{\text{kg}}{2.2\text{ lb}} \times \frac{40\text{ mg}}{\text{kg} \times \text{day}} = 800\text{ mg/day}$$

$$\text{Prescribed Daily Dose: } \frac{10\text{ mL}}{6\text{ hours}} \times \frac{100\text{ mg}}{5\text{ mL}} \times \frac{24\text{ hours}}{\text{day}} = 800\text{ mg/day}$$

89. D. Sterile compounding.

To review sterile compounding, see pages 213 – 224.

90. B. Darkness

To review storage considerations, see pages 144 – 146.

91. C. 9.9 mL

$$\frac{2.1\text{ mL of Alcohol}}{100\text{ mL of Cheratussin}^{®}\text{ DAC}} \times 473\text{ mL of Cheratussin}^{®}\text{ DAC} = 9.9\text{ mL of Alcohol}$$

To review percent concentration calculations, see pages 179 – 180.

92. A. 30 minutes

To review this topic, see page 219.

93. A. 0.22 microns

To review this topic, see page 220.

94. B. 2 pairs

To review procedures for handling hazardous drugs, see pages 227 – 229.

95. C. 84 days

$$12 \text{ capsules} \times \frac{\text{week}}{1 \text{ capsule}} \times \frac{7 \text{ days}}{\text{week}} = 84 \text{ days}$$

96. C. 67 drops/minute

$$100 \text{ mL} \times \frac{20 \text{ drops}}{\text{mL}} \times \frac{1}{30 \text{ minutes}} = 67 \text{ drops/minute}$$

To review IV drip rate calculations, see pages 205 – 207.

97. B. 31 gauge, 12.7 millimeters

$$0.5 \text{ inch} \times \frac{2.54 \text{ cm}}{\text{inch}} \times \frac{10 \text{ millimeters}}{\text{cm}} = 12.7 \text{ millimeters}$$

To review gauge sizes, see page 222. To review the Must-Know Conversion Factors, see page 163.

98. C. In red ink, the letter "C" at least 1 inch high.

CONTROLLED SUBSTANCE PRESCRIPTION RECORDS	
C-II:	Must keep separate from all other prescriptions.
C-III, C-IV, & C-V:	Keep separate from all other prescriptions, or mark in the lower right corner with the letter "C" at least 1-inch high in red ink and store in the same file with non-controlled substance prescriptions.

To review the summary of controlled substance laws, see page 40.

99. D. Viagra® + Nitrostat®

To review common drug interactions, see pages 123 – 125.

100. C. Joint inflammation

"**Arthr-**" means joint; "**-itis**" means inflammation.

To review medical terminology word parts, see pages 12 – 13.

101. B. Action word, quantity with units, route of administration, dosing frequency

To review prescription sigs, see page 131.

102. B. A few days

To this topic, see page 150.

103. D. A drug product can only be compounded after receiving an individual, patient-specific prescription order, or in anticipation of receiving a patient-specific prescription order based on an established prescribing pattern.

To review compounding, see page 173.

104. B. Artificial nails

To review this topic, see page 214.

105. B. 4 ounces

CXX = 120

$$120 \text{ mL} \times \frac{\text{ounce}}{30 \text{ mL}} = 4 \text{ ounces}$$

To review Roman numerals, see pages 153 – 154.

106. A. Schedule II

To review controlled substances categorized by schedule, see pages 32 – 35.

107. C. CMS

To review this topic, see page 149.

108. A. Premium

Deductibles and co-payments are only paid when the insurance is used. Premiums are paid to maintain active coverage, regardless of whether the patient is using the insurance. To review this topic further, see page 148.

109. C. Drugs for pain

To review key terms, see pages 14 – 21.

110. B. Novolin 70/30

BRAND NAME	GENERIC NAME	
Humulin R®, Novolin R®	Regular Human Insulin	OTC
Humulin N®, Novolin N®	Insulin NPH	
Novolin 70/30®, Humulin 70/30®	Mixture of 70% Insulin NPH and 30% Regular Human Insulin	

To review the section on insulin, see page 91.

111. A. Vitamin K

To review this topic, see page 125.

112. B. 28 days

Insulin vials expire after 28 days at room temperature and/or once the rubber stopper of the vial is punctured. To review insulin, see page 91.

113. A. Toprol XL® - III. Metoprolol (ER)
B. Lamisil® - II. Terbinafine
C. Ritalin® - IV. Methylphenidate
D. Apresoline® - V. Hydralazine
E. Tegretol® - I. Carbamazepine

To review the top 200 prescription drugs, see pages 116 – 120.

114. B. 56 capsules

$$\frac{1 \text{ capsule}}{6 \text{ hours}} \times \frac{24 \text{ hours}}{\text{day}} \times \frac{14 \text{ days}}{1} = 56 \text{ capsules}$$

115. D. 240 mEq

$$\frac{\text{mEq} \times \text{Molecular Weight}}{\text{Valence}} = ?\ \text{mg} \qquad \frac{12 \text{ mEq} \times 40}{2} = 240 \text{ mg}$$

To review milliequivalents, see pages 171 – 172.

116. C. Enforce federal controlled substance laws.

To review the role of government agencies, see page 51.

117. D. Evaluate prescriptions for drug interactions.

To review this topic, see pages 23 – 24.

118. B. 227 g of Eucerin® cream and 227 g of triamcinolone 0.5% ointment

The prescription asks for a one-pound mixture containing equal parts of Eucerin® cream and triamcinolone 0.5% ointment. This is a simple unit conversion problem. We already know that we need one-half pound of each ingredient. The question is really just asking how many grams are in one-half pound. You must have the conversion factor committed to memory; there are 454 grams in 1 pound. One-half of 454 grams is 227 grams. Therefore, to compound this prescription you will need 227 grams of Eucerin® cream and 227 grams of triamcinolone 0.5% ointment. If your answer was incorrect, you need to go back to page 163 and memorize the Must-Know Conversion Factors.

119. B. Apply to affected area twice daily as needed for itchy rash

To review prescription sigs, see pages 131 – 135.

120. C. 18 years old

To review OTC Schedule V controlled substance sales, see page 41.

$$\% \text{ Error} = \frac{\text{Sensitivity Requirement}}{\text{Desired Weight}} \times 100\%$$

$$\text{Density} = \frac{\text{Mass (grams)}}{\text{Volume (milliliters)}}$$

$$\text{Specific Gravity} = \frac{\text{Density of Substance}}{\text{Density of Reference Substance}}$$

$$°\text{C} = \frac{5}{9}\,(°\text{F} - 32)$$

$$°\text{F} = \left(\frac{9}{5} \times °\text{C}\right) + 32$$

$$\text{BSA} = \sqrt{\frac{\text{height (cm)} \times \text{weight (kg)}}{3{,}600}}$$

$$\text{Child Dose (Clark's Rule)} = \frac{\text{Weight (lb)}}{150 \text{ lb}} \times \text{Adult Dose}$$

$$\text{Child Dose (Young's Rule)} = \frac{\text{Age}}{(\text{Age} + 12)} \times \text{Adult Dose}$$

$$\text{Child Dose (BSA Dosing)} = \frac{\text{BSA}}{1.73 \text{ m}^2} \times \text{Adult Dose}$$

$$\frac{\text{mg} \times \text{Valence}}{\text{Molecular Weight}} = \text{mEq}$$

$$\frac{\text{mEq} \times \text{Molecular Weight}}{\text{Valence}} = \text{mg}$$

Retail Cost = [AWP x (1 + Markup*)] + Dispensing Fee
*Markup expressed as a decimal

JOHN
3:16

Made in United States
Troutdale, OR
08/28/2025

34049354R00156